HANDBOOK OF
NITROUS OXIDE AND OXYGEN SEDATION

HANDBOOK OF

NITROUS OXIDE AND OXYGEN SEDATION

MORRIS CLARK, DDS, FACD

Professor, Oral and Maxillofacial Surgery
Director of Anesthesia
Department of Surgical Dentistry, School of Dentistry
Professor of Surgery, School of Medicine
University of Colorado Health Sciences Center
Denver, Colorado

ANN BRUNICK, RDH, MS

Chairperson and Professor
Department of Dental Hygiene
University of South Dakota
Vermillion, South Dakota

Second Edition

With 124 illustrations

An Affiliate of Elsevier Science

Mosby

An Affiliate of Elsevier Science

11830 Westline Industrial Drive
St. Louis, Missouri 63146

HANDBOOK OF NITROUS OXIDE AND   ISBN 0-323-01977-3
OXYGEN SEDATION
Copyright © 2003, Mosby, Inc. All rights reserved.

Previous edition copyrighted 1999

Library of Congress Cataloging in Publication Data
Clark, Morris
    Handbook of nitrous oxide and oxygen sedation / Morris Shandell Clark, Ann Brunick.–2nd ed.
      p. ; cm.
    Includes bibliographical references and index.
    ISBN 0-323-01977-3
    1. Nitrous oxide–Therapeutic use–Handbooks, manuals, etc. 2. Oxygen therapy–Handbooks, manuals, etc. 3. Anesthesia in dentistry–Handbooks, manuals, etc. 4. Conscious sedation–Handbooks, manuals, etc. 5. Inhalation anesthesia–Handbooks, manuals, etc. I. Brunick, Ann L. II. Title.
    [DNLM: 1. Nitrous Oxide–therapeutic use–Handbooks. 2. Anesthesia, Inhalation–Handbooks. 3. Conscious Sedation–Handbooks. 4. Oxygen–therapeutic use–Handbooks. QV 39 C594h 2003]
    RK512.N55C58 2003
    617.9'676–dc21   2003044196

Publishing Director: Linda L. Duncan
Executive Editor: Penny Rudolph
Developmental Editor: Jaime Pendill
Publishing Services Manager: Linda McKinley
Project Manager: Jennifer Furey
Designer: Gail Morey Hudson

Printed in the United States of America

Last digit is the print number: 9   8   7   6   5   4   3   2   1

To my mother,
Clarie Clark *(1910-2002),*
who taught me humor and perseverance
MSC

To
Paul, Adam, and **Kyle,**
with gratitude for their love and support
ALB

FOREWORD

The intimate association of nitrous oxide inhalation and dentistry has existed for approximately 150 years. The advantages of administering nitrous oxide and oxygen sedation during dental procedures are many. It is very safe. It is pleasantly received by patients. It produces a rapid and deep analgesia while leaving the patient cooperative. It is quickly eliminated by the body, allowing the patient to return to baseline without lingering side effects. Nitrous oxide continues to be an integral part of dental practice today. It is estimated that more than 50% of general dentists and nearly 90% of pediatric dentists administer it to their patients to alleviate procedural anxiety and pain. It was quite natural, then, that two dental professionals—Dr. Morris Clark, a professor of oral and maxillofacial surgery, and Ann Brunick, a professor of dental hygiene—would collaborate to give us the *Handbook of Nitrous Oxide and Oxygen Sedation*, now in an expanded and reorganized second edition.

The second edition is broad in scope, and I would recommend it to healthcare practitioners of any discipline responsible for patients requiring sedation for unpleasant procedures. Appropriately, the core of the book describes the scientific principles, clinical indications, and practical techniques for administering nitrous oxide and oxygen. The authors' thorough descriptions of patient evaluation, pre-procedure preparation, and monitoring are applicable to all forms of sedation. They also discuss effective communication skills and advocate for the ethical and compassionate treatment of patients. Every practitioner involved in the administration of sedation would benefit by becoming familiar with the information covered in this book.

Two new chapters in this edition are especially notable. Chapter One, *Practice Guidelines*, refers to two sets of guidelines, one established by the American Society of Anesthesiologists (ASA) and the other by the American Dental Association (ADA). *Practice Guidelines for Sedation and Analgesia by Non-Anesthesiologists* was originally adopted by the ASA in 1995 and was revised in 2002. *Guidelines for the Use of Conscious Sedation, Deep Sedation and General Anesthesia for Dentists* was adopted by the ADA in 2002. These guidelines were intended to help practitioners who are not specialists in anesthesiology provide their patients with anxiety and pain control during diagnostic or therapeutic procedures. Neither of these documents was designed to cover minimal sedation (anxiolysis) since it entails minimal risk. Minimal sedation includes situations where nitrous oxide is used in concentrations of less than 50%, either alone or with local anesthesia. The guidelines are applicable when more than

50% nitrous oxide is administered, or when nitrous oxide is given in combination with other sedatives. The guidelines give valuable recommendations regarding patient evaluation, monitoring, and recovery care. Both the ASA and the ADA emphasize that sedative drugs should be titrated, that is, given in small incremental doses to achieve optimal effect. Clark and Brunick also advocate for the titration method of administering nitrous oxide.

Another notable inclusion in this edition is Chapter 16, *Clinical Application of Nitrous Oxide and Oxygen Sedation in Pediatrics.* When performing painful procedures on children, practitioners can easily inflict long-lasting emotional injuries if they fail to adequately address a child's anxiety and need for pain control. Children are typically accepting of inhalation sedation since it does not involve placing an intravenous catheter, and in fact, the majority of pediatric dentists use nitrous oxide in their practice. Clark and Brunick suggest that patients who have had positive healthcare experiences during childhood may be more likely to behave positively toward healthcare providers in the future. By treating them in a humane fashion during diagnostic and therapeutic procedures, practitioners can greatly attenuate the emotional scars that children might otherwise bear for a lifetime.

I have worked with Dr. Clark for a number of years in the operating room. He is compassionate and meticulous in his practice, and his writing conveys these same qualities. With their second edition of the *Handbook of Nitrous Oxide and Oxygen Sedation*, Dr. Clark and Ann Brunick have bestowed on us a guide for the safe administration of nitrous oxide and a model for humane patient care.

David R. Theil, MD
Medical Director, Department of Anesthesia
Rose Medical Center
Denver, Colorado

PREFACE

The second edition of this text is written with the knowledge that our first edition is now ready for an update. We have had the opportunity to clarify some concepts and illustrate them better, as well as the opportunity to enhance the literature in the area of sedation using nitrous oxide and oxygen. There is a great measure of pride in knowing that our first attempt was so universally received. It exceeded our publisher's expectations and, more importantly, crossed several health professional disciplines. Our intent remains the same: to provide a concise, user-friendly text in an outline format that is not an unnecessarily burdensome reference on nitrous oxide/oxygen sedation.

During this revision process, we were guided by the recently published updated guidelines from the American Society of Anesthesiology entitled *Practice Guidelines for Sedation and Analgesia by Non-Anesthesiologists.* It serves as the standard of care for nitrous oxide/oxygen sedation.

We have had the privilege to lecture throughout the United States and the world on nitrous oxide/oxygen sedation and have recorded suggestions and information that we sincerely hope improve the quality of this text. Of particular note is the fact that this text was translated into the Polish language and subsequently has received a wide acclaim for a large segment of practitioners who now use this method of pain and anxiety management. We could not be happier or more honored.

A distinctive feature of the second edition is a new chapter solely devoted to pediatrics. There is also a new chapter that provides answers to frequently asked questions about nitrous oxide/oxygen sedation. This edition includes the most accurate information regarding the issue of biohazards and an updated literature review. In addition, the most recent equipment available for sedation delivery is illustrated in this clinically oriented text.

We continue to be impressed with the amazing fact that an American dentist, Dr. Horace Wells, the father of anesthesia, made such an enduring contribution to mankind. We believe the interest in nitrous oxide/oxygen sedation has never been higher and that the enthusiasm and faith in its ability to provide effective pain and anxiety management for patients has not wavered, but rather increased. This textbook is the most popular reference on nitrous oxide/oxygen sedation across the health disciplines and we believe it is a significant contribution to the body of scientific knowledge and the advancement of education in this area. As information emerges in the literature and safe administration and monitoring techniques are practiced in clinical settings, we are indeed encouraged about the future of pain and anxiety management using nitrous oxide and oxygen.

Morris Clark, DDS, FACD
Ann Brunick, RDH, MS

ACKNOWLEDGMENTS

We would like to acknowledge all the supporters of this second edition of the *Handbook of Nitrous Oxide and Oxygen Sedation*.

We owe a great deal to the manufacturers of nitrous oxide/oxygen sedation equipment that have not only graciously contributed to this text, but, more importantly, have also cooperated with one another and the dental community to provide the very best equipment possible for our patients. Thank you for your dedication and professionalism. They are, in alphabetical order, Accutron, Inc. of Phoenix, AZ; MDS Matrx of Orchard Park, NY; and Porter Instrument Company, Inc. of Hatfield, PA. In particular, we appreciate consultation from Mr. Jonathan Blaisdell, Mr. Chris Wilson, and Mr. Dan Shoemaker.

We are grateful for the tireless effort of Dr. Janusz Kacki for his true dedication in bringing the Polish translation from initiation to fruition. He is truly an incredible practitioner.

Special thanks go to Ms. Celia Zermatten, Dr. Carlos Plateroti, and Dr. Stanley Malamed.

Several individuals from the University of Colorado Health Sciences Center deserve thanks for their support. They are Dean Howard Landesman, Dr. Donald Kleier, Dr. James Lindenmuth, Dr. Mike Savage, and Ms. Debbie Malley.

Others to thank include Dr. Will Miles, Mr. Willie Clark, Dr. Boyd Tomasetti, Dr. Peter Steinhauer, Dr. Mark Gillman, Ms. Mercedes Merchant, Mr. Dan Chemsak, Ms. Jan Connolly, Ms. Laura Woodruff, Ms. Vanessa Hernandez, Dr. Mort Rosenberg, Dr. Elizabeth Barr, and Dr. Steve Wilson.

Individuals from the University of South Dakota that deserve thanks are Mr. Glen Malchow, Ms. Erin DeJong, Ms. Leslie Byers, Ms. Christina Fincham, Ms. Cassie Thiewes, Ms. Christy Dunlop, Mr. Romney Jones, Ms. Bev Murra, and Ms. Beverly Kennedy.

Finally, we would like to offer special thanks to Ms. Penny Rudolph, Executive Editor at Mosby, Inc., for her unending support. In addition, we are grateful to Ms. Jaime Pendill for her assistance in helping us publish this manuscript in a timely manner.

CONTENTS

PART I INTRODUCTION TO NITROUS OXIDE/OXYGEN SEDATION, I

1   Practice Guidelines, 3

2   History and Evolution of N_2O/O_2 Sedation, 6

3   Pain and Anxiety Management, 16

4   Comparison of N_2O/O_2 Sedation to Other Sedation Methods, 28

5   Physical Properties and Pharmacokinetics of N_2O, 33

6   Manufacturing and Distribution of N_2O and O_2 Gases, 41

7   Economic Benefits Associated with N_2O/O_2 Administration, 70

PART II ANATOMY, PHYSIOLOGY, AND ADMINISTRATION, 75

8   Anatomy and Physiology of Respiration and Airway Management, 77

9   N_2O and its Interaction with the Body, 89

10 Patient Assessment, 99

11 Titration of N_2O/O_2 Gases, 107

12 Signs and Symptoms of N_2O/O_2 Sedation, 111

13 Technique for N_2O/O_2 Administration, 118

14 Recovery from N_2O/O_2 Sedation, 144

15 Multidisciplinary Application of N_2O/O_2 Sedation, 149

16 Clinical Application of N_2O/O_2 Sedation in Pediatrics, 163

PART III ISSUES OF SPECIAL CONSIDERATION, 169

17 Potential Biohazards for Health Personnel Associated with Chronic Exposure to N_2O, 171

18 N_2O Abuse Issues, 185

19   Ethical and Legal Considerations Regarding N_2O Administration, 197

20   Commonly Asked Questions Regarding N_2O/O_2 Sedation, 201

21   Future Trends in N_2O/O_2 Sedation, 204

APPENDIXES, 205
A   Manufacturers and Organizational Resources, 207
B   Percent of N_2O/O_2 Administered, 212
C N_2O/O_2 Sedation Record, 214
D   Informed Consent for N_2O/O_2 Sedation, 215
E   Overview of Administration of N_2O/O_2 Sedation, 216
F   Health Insurance Portability and Accountability Act (HIPAA) of 1996, 217
G   Overview of CDC Hand Hygiene Guidelines, 220

HANDBOOK OF
NITROUS OXIDE AND OXYGEN SEDATION

PART I

INTRODUCTION TO NITROUS OXIDE/OXYGEN SEDATION

I
Practice Guidelines

Before the "greatest discovery of all time," surgical procedures required people to endure horrific experiences that were, at best, tenuous in therapeutic benefit and too often resulted in death. This was in spite of skilled, dedicated practitioners who risked their own lives to advance the cure or alter the direction of a disease process.[1] Since its discovery more than 150 years ago, nitrous oxide (N_2O) has been used to provide pain and anxiety relief for patients undergoing surgical procedures.[2] More than 24 million surgical procedures are performed each year in the United States,[2] and in a large number of them, nitrous oxide/oxygen (N_2O/O_2) in combination with other drugs is used to facilitate general anesthesia.

In addition to its use as a general anesthetic adjuvant, myriad health disciplines use N_2O/O_2 sedation alone as an effective means of alleviating patient anxiety and mild discomfort during ambulatory and outpatient procedures. For the patient, N_2O/O_2 provides pain control and anxiety relief that is quickly and easily reversed with minimal side effects. For the practitioner, the drug is easily titrated to the level required for the procedure while accommodating the patient's physiologic and psychologic needs. Nitrous oxide has been cited extensively in the literature for more than 150 years as a safe and effective drug. Most of the early literature refers to dentistry as the discipline that first acknowledged the anesthetic potential of N_2O. Nitrous oxide is notable because of its impeccable safety record, which has withstood the test of time longer than any other drug. Gardner Quincy Colton (1864-1897), an itinerant professor, documented 193,000 cases with no adverse reactions.[3] Ruben,[4] a Danish researcher, cites 3,000,000 cases using N_2O/O_2 in the dental office with no adverse reactions noted. Niels Bjorn Jorgensen[5] attests to 4,000,000 episodes without complications.

When used as a mild analgesic and sedative, N_2O is administered with oxygen from safe modern equipment that allows no more than 70% N_2O and no less than 30% O_2 to be delivered at any time. The patient is mildly sedated and responds to verbal commands. Protective defenses such as the cough and gag reflexes remain intact; clinical action and elimination are rapid. Recovery is complete within a short time. There are few side effects associated with N_2O, provided the operator uses updated equipment and an appropriate technique. Most often, patients' negative experiences with N_2O have been caused by oversedation by the operator. To that end, this text will emphasize the titration aspect of the administration technique.

Current Practice Guidelines

Recently a metaanalysis entitled "Practice Guidelines for Sedation and Analgesia by Non-Anesthesiologists" was published in *Anesthesiology*.[6] These guidelines, developed by the American Society of Anesthesiology (ASA), serve as the overriding policy for defining and directing the trends and practice of N_2O/O_2 administration into the foreseeable future.[6] The guidelines are meant to direct those who are *not* specialists in anesthesiology and they are mandatory for nonanesthesiologists practicing in hospitals (e.g., physicians, dentists, podiatrists, etc.). They are clearly useful and set the standard of care for future practice. We will refer to them throughout this text because the guidelines represent an extensive evaluation (36-year electronic search and 44-year manual search) and a synthesis of expert opinion by numerous academic and clinical anesthesiologists across the United States.

To support the ASA practice guidelines, we will also refer to the recent document from the American Dental Association (ADA).[7] In October 2002, the ADA House of Delegates adopted the "Guidelines for the Use of Conscious Sedation, Deep Sedation and General Anesthesia for Dentists."[7] Included in these guidelines for the first time is the term *titration* and its definition. Although the guidelines are not intended for anxiolysis produced by N_2O/O_2 alone, they do refer to the use of N_2O/O_2 in combination with other pharmacologic methods when conscious (moderate) sedation is intended.

This text focuses on the use of N_2O/O_2 in an ambulatory setting. Much of the literature relates to the use of N_2O as an adjunct anesthetic in the operating room for general anesthesia; therefore, reference will be made to articles in the literature in that setting. However, when N_2O/O_2 is used in the ambulatory setting, it is used for minimal periods of time and with lower percentage concentrations. The ASA *Practice Guidelines for Sedation and Analgesia by Non-Anesthesiologists* do not address minimal sedation or anxiolysis, which is the administration of N_2O in concentrations less than 50%. The guidelines exclude minimal sedation because at this level of sedation the risks are minimal and adverse effects are negligible. Occasionally, the practitioner may apply N_2O in concentrations greater than 50%. For this reason, we will also address the ASA task force recommendations for moderate sedation because this is the category in which administration of N_2O in concentrations greater than 50% is placed. In this document, the term *conscious sedation* has been replaced with the updated term *moderate sedation*. There are specific levels of responsibility for the nonanesthesiologist when a patient is sedated at this level. *The guidelines recommend that the practitioner be responsible for the patient at the intended level of sedation and the next (deeper) level of sedation.* This concept is clearly based on the practitioner being thoroughly educated and trained, thereby increasing the safety margin for the patient. In this edition of the text, we include recommendations for managing moderate sedation and management of the airway. Nitrous oxide-oxygen sedation is still simple and safe to use.

Use of N₂O/O₂

N_2O/O_2 sedation may not provide the desired results for all practitioners, nor will it be an option for all patients. However, it continues to maintain its position for effective pain and anxiety management.

REFERENCES

1. Smith WDA: *Under the influence: a history of nitrous oxide and oxygen anesthesia*, Park Ridge, Ill, 1982, Wood Library, Museum of Anesthesiology.
2. Kole T: Assessing the potential for awareness and learning under anesthesia, *J Am Assoc Nurse Anes* 61:571, 1993.
3. Chancellor JW: Dr. Wells' impact on dentistry and medicine, *J Am Dent Assoc* 125:1585, 1994.
4. Ruben H: Nitrous oxide analgesia in dentistry, *Br Dent J* 132:195, 1972.
5. Jorgensen NB: Sedation, local and general anesthesia in dentistry, ed 2, Philadelphia, 1985, Lea & Febiger.
6. ASA Task Force: Practice guidelines for sedation and analgesia by non-anesthesiologists, *Anesthesiology* 96(4):1004, 2002.
7. American Dental Association: Guidelines for the use of conscious sedation, deep sedation, and general anesthesia for dentists, ADA House of Delegates, October 2002, American Dental Association.

2
History and Evolution of N_2O/O_2 Sedation

In this era of sophisticated medicine and high technology it is easy to forget what early medical scientists went through to advance standard practices such as N_2O/O_2 sedation. What these scientific pioneers accomplished while experimenting with unknown, potentially dangerous materials and primitive equipment is amazing. They often sacrificed their own health and safety for the sake of scientific advancement. It is because of the tenacity of these early medical explorers that we can provide safe and effective analgesia and anesthesia today.

I. Historical Perspectives

A. Discovery of N_2O and O_2
  1. The discovery of both N_2O and O_2 is credited to the English gentleman, Joseph Priestley.
  2. The actual discovery dates of these gases are somewhat in question because of Priestley's own uncertainty about what he had discovered. The periods cited in the literature vary from 1771 to 1777.[1] During this time he repeated several experiments that ultimately resulted in the gases we know today as N_2O and O_2.
  3. Priestley experimented with nitrous air—a mixture of iron filings, sulfur, and water. The end product was a residual gas with considerably less volume than the original nitrous air. He called this "dephlogisticated nitrous air," which is now known as nitrous oxide.[1]
  4. During his experiments with nitrous air, Priestly became aware of another gas, which he termed "good air." He found this air to be "fit for respiration," and he titled this discovery "dephlogisticated air," which is now known as oxygen.[1]
B. Inhalation of N_2O
  1. Humphrey Davy, at the age of 21, was interested in the field of medicine. Although N_2O gas was allegedly etiologic to many diseases and deadly conditions, Davy ignored the warnings and, in England in 1798, became the first to chronically inhale pure N_2O.
  2. Instead of incurring some dreadful plight, Davy found the experience very pleasurable; he became euphoric and felt like laughing. He continued his experiments, saying they produced the "most voluptuous sensations." Other descriptions of his experiences with N_2O included "ideal

existence" and "overwhelming joy."[2] Davy published the results of his experiments in booklet form in 1800.

3. It was when Davy experienced diminished pain from a toothache while using N_2O that he began to believe it could affect pain sensations. This was the first indication of the anesthetic properties of the gas. Davy had no idea of the significance of this experience.

4. For the next four decades, experiments with N_2O continued, but not in the medical field. Nineteen-year-old Samuel Colt (of firearm fame), posing as a physician, began sporting street corner sideshows featuring N_2O. These shows were touted as a way for young people to enjoy evening entertainment during which they could "laugh, sing, speak, or fight."[3] N_2O use became the trendy activity at social events and in university settings (Figures 2-1 and 2-2). It was the featured demonstration at many lectures.

Laughing Gas.

Figure 2-1 "Laughing Gas." (From Scoffern: *Chemistry No Mystery*, 1839. Courtesy of the Harvard Medical Library in the F.A. Countway Library of Medicine, Boston, Mass.)

Figure 2-2   Poster advertising a nitrous oxide exhibition. (From Malamed SF: *Sedation*, ed 4, St Louis, 2003, Mosby.)

     5. The anesthetic value of N_2O first realized by Davy was not pursued.

C. Medical world ignores N_2O as potential anesthetic

     1. During the early nineteenth century, while reckless use of N_2O continued, the medical community was hungry for pain relief. Surgical procedures often resulted in death of patients for many reasons. Poor infection control often led to secondary infections and the lack of pain control was problematic.

     2. The most commonly performed operations were amputations, tooth extractions, and abscess draining. These surgeries were completed within minutes and often in less than 90 seconds. However, during more lengthy procedures patients would succumb to exhaustion and/or shock.

     3. The greatest medical advance at that time was the suture. Wounds could be sewn closed rather than cauterized with a hot iron; extremities remaining from amputations did not have to be dipped in a boiling solution to cause hemostasis.[3]

4. Prospective patients often committed suicide rather than face an operation without pain control. Pain control measures were time-consuming, unpredictable, inconsistent, and at best mildly effective. Several methods were tried.
   a. Brute force to hold a patient down
   b. Preoperative alcohol or opium
   c. Tourniquets, ice, and hypnotism

5. Obviously, prospective surgical patients were often placed in serious dilemmas—choosing between pure torture and unfathomable pain associated with surgery or living with a disease or condition that would more than likely result in a slow, agonizing death.

D. The revelation at Dr. Colton's Grand Exhibition

1. Dr. Gardner Colton, a Columbia University dropout turned professor, hosted the Grand Exhibition in Hartford, Connecticut on December 10, 1844. It was an exhibition to demonstrate the exhilarating effects of inhaling N_2O.[4]

2. Horace Wells, a dentist, was in attendance. As a participant, Wells volunteered to try the gas on stage, believing he would not "make a spectacle of himself." However, that was exactly how Mrs. Wells described his performance.[2]

3. Another participant, a young man named Samuel Cooley, volunteered to inhale the gas in front of the audience. He began to feel the effects of the gas immediately. As he was euphorically jumping around, he hit his leg against a bench, causing a deep, bloody laceration. Cooley was unaware of the extent of the injury and professed that he did not feel any pain.

4. Wells was very intrigued by the apparent nonresponsiveness of Cooley to pain and asked Colton whether a tooth could be removed under the influence of N_2O. Unaware of any analgesic properties, Colton agreed to bring a supply of gas and meet Wells at his office the next day. There Wells breathed the gas himself and had a colleague, Dr. Riggs, extract one of his teeth. Wells exclaimed "the greatest discovery ever made," and "a new era in tooth pulling." Colton taught Wells how to prepare the N_2O and thought of him as a "visionary enthusiast."[4] Figure 2-3 shows a one-of-a-kind portrait of Wells that appears at the Wadsworth Antheneum in Hartford, Connecticut.

E. The Horace Wells experiment

1. Wells used N_2O during extractions on several patients with great success. Anxious to demonstrate this procedure in front of his peers, Wells was allowed to operate in front of several physicians and students in Boston in 1845. As he attempted to remove a tooth, the patient jumped in the chair, leading observers to believe he was in pain. Some time later the patient indicated he did not experience any pain.[4] Unfortunately for Wells, his experiment was deemed unsuccessful and he was labeled a "charlatan" and a "fake."[5]

2. Wells, in his own writings, indicated that he was obsessed with proving the legitimacy of his techniques. He also alluded to being severely depressed over the debacle in Boston.[5]

Figure 2-3   Portrait of Dr. Horace Wells, Discoverer of Anesthesia. (Wadsworth Antheneum, Hartford. Gift of Charles Nöel Flagg. Endowed by C.N. Flagg and Company.)

3. For the next several years Wells continued to provide anesthesia for surgeons in the area. Dentists began to give attention to the use of N_2O. In fact, advancing dentistry's reputation hinged on the success of extracting teeth with pain relief.[6]

II. Evolution of Anesthesia

A. Ether anesthesia
  1. William Morton, a dental student of Wells' and later a physician, was present at the famed event presented by Wells in Boston. Believing that a more potent anesthetic gas was necessary, he began to work with ether.
  2. In 1846, Morton performed a surgical demonstration using ether in the Massachusetts General Hospital, later called the "ether dome" (Figure 2-4). Morton's experiment was similar to Wells' in terms of poor success; the patient stated that he felt the procedure as it was performed. However, the demonstration was well received by the audience primarily because of Morton's status as a physician rather than a dentist.[7]
  3. Surgical procedures using ether continued. Other individuals claiming to be the discoverer of anesthesia led Morton to fight for recognition.

Figure 2-4   The "Ether Dome" present (1997). (Photo courtesy of Dr. Peter Jacobsohn.)

Morton died tragically in 1848 never having been officially recognized for his accomplishments.

B. Chloroform anesthesia
   1. In 1847, English obstetrician James Simpson was pleased with the anesthetic properties of ether for his patients. However, he did not like the odor or its potential to induce vomiting. He began to use chloroform as an analgesic for labor pains despite others' claims of significant negative consequences.[6]
   2. Chloroform continued to be a major anesthetic agent into the 1860s and became standard issue to soldiers who, when injured in battle, could self-administer it.[3]
C. The fight for recognition
   1. After his failed performance using N_2O as an anesthetic, Wells' whereabouts and mental status were uncertain for a few years. It was very important to him that he prove his credibility and be recognized for his accomplishments. Although the concept of addiction was not recognized at that time, Wells had become a chloroform addict with unpredictable behavior. Inhaling chloroform contributed to his mental decline and, while in a stupor, Wells threw acid on a prostitute in New York City and was imprisoned in 1848. He asked to retrieve some personal items from his home and brought a razor and some chloroform back to his cell. He wrote his last words to his wife and committed suicide by cutting his femoral artery while under the influence of the drug. He died at the age of 33, unaware of the credit being given to him while serving his sentence.[5]
   2. The Medical Society of Paris, France was the first to grant Wells "all the honors of having first discovered and successfully applied the uses of

vapors or gases whereby operations could be performed without pain"[4] (Figure 2-5).

3. In Hartford, Connecticut, every physician had signed a document proclaiming Wells as the primary discoverer of anesthesia.[8]

4. In 1864, the American Dental Association (ADA) officially recognized him, and in 1870 the American Medical Association (AMA) proclaimed this honor. Reaffirmation was proclaimed by the AMA on the one hundredth anniversary (1944) of the original exhibition, and in the sesquicentennial year (1994) several dental and anesthesiology societies affirmed once again Wells' significant contributions to the health professions.[8] Also in 1994, he was posthumously awarded the Doctor of Dental Surgery degree from the Baltimore College of Dentistry, the first school of dentistry in the United States.

5. In addition, Dr. Leonard F. Menszer led a nationwide petition for a commemorative postage stamp (Figure 2-6).[9] Unfortunately, despite thousands of signatures, the stamp has yet to be issued.

6. The Horace Wells Club, an organization of dentists and physicians, was formed in 1897 in Hartford, Connecticut on the fiftieth anniversary of Wells' discovery. They have been meeting for the last 107 years to remember this great benefactor and foster the study of anesthesiology. The Horace Wells Club also sponsors scholarships for dental students from

Figure 2-5   Bust of Horace Wells in the Etats Unis Park near the Arc de Triomphe in Paris, France (2002).

Figure 2-6   Petition for commemorative stamp, 1994. (Photo courtesy of Dr. Peter Jacobsohn.)

Connecticut and they restore and maintain the statue of Horace Wells in Hartford's Bushnell Park. They also present an award of merit annually to an individual who has demonstrated leadership and achievement in the field of sedation.[10]

D. Resurgence of N_2O

1. The same Dr. Colton who supplied Wells with N_2O in 1844 was responsible for its resurfacing in the early 1860s. Colton insisted that pure N_2O was safe and had an impeccable record of cases to prove it. Between 1864 and 1897 Colton documented 193,000 cases with no fatalities.[6] This began the establishment of its safety record.

2. In 1868, Dr. Edmund Andrews suggested that, when 100% N_2O is used, the blood is not appropriately oxygenated. Andrews added O_2 to the N_2O and claimed one fifth of the volume should be O_2.[2]

3. Also in 1868, Paul Bert developed equipment to deliver both O_2 and N_2O to a patient.[11] He recommended greater atmospheric pressure when using N_2O/O_2 for human surgeries. However, although his idea was ingenious, it was impractical because of the size and relative immobility of the associated equipment.

E. Twentieth century

1. Dentistry continued to be the primary health discipline to use N_2O. However, except for episodic periods between 1913 and 1938, N_2O use

was almost nonexistent. Reasons for this inactivity were unreliable equipment, failure to produce satisfactory results, and lack of knowledge of technique.

2. Cyclopropane was discovered in 1929 and was subsequently used in the clinical setting as a general anesthetic. An excellent anesthetic, it remained the most popular agent for general anesthesia for the next 30 years; its use declined because of flammability issues.[7]

3. Medical residencies in the 1930s included N_2O information in their curricula. Anesthesia became a specialty in 1941.[6] Dr. Harry Langa, an early proponent of N_2O/O_2, began postgraduate dental education in 1949 and trained more than 6000 dentists in N_2O sedation. Dr. Langa also published a classic textbook on N_2O inhalation analgesia.[2]

4. Physicians were not satisfied with the availability and effectiveness of intravenous (IV) agents until sodium thiopental (barbiturate) was deemed acceptable in 1935.[7]

5. Curare was used by anesthesiologists in the 1940s to provide muscle relaxation with light levels of sedation during surgery. When curare was used with N_2O, the incidences of mortality and morbidity were decreased. This combination became the anesthetic of choice for high-risk patients because it did not threaten the cardiovascular system.[7]

6. The 1940s also brought the discovery of local anesthesia to dentistry, which revolutionized pain control in that setting.[12] The popularity and acceptance of local anesthesia temporarily diminished the use of N_2O. When the role of N_2O was revised to assist with the management of anxiety, its popularity began to rise again.

7. The nonflammable anesthetic agent halothane was introduced in 1956.[7] This introduced a whole new era of anesthetic techniques. Halothane was highly regarded in the medical community because of the minimal side effects associated with its use. This offered a great improvement over other general anesthetics at the time. N_2O was used as an adjuvant drug to induce the effects of halothane.

8. N_2O remained functional and was commonly used for general anesthesia as a way to provide rapid induction of other more potent agents.

9. Dental schools began teaching the concepts of inhalation sedation in the late 1950s and early 1960s. In 1962, guidelines for teaching pain and anxiety control in dentistry were established by the American Dental Society of Anesthesiology. Today this organization remains at the cutting edge, helping to develop new drugs, techniques, and training for dentists in the area of anesthesia. Also, the International Federation of Dental Anesthesia Societies (IFDAS) is an organization composed of component societies from around the globe. They convene every 3 years to present the latest in scientific data and exchange research findings for the promotion of pain and anxiety control. N_2O continues to be popular in the field of dentistry; approximately 56% of general dentists, 85% of oral and maxillofacial surgeons, and 88% of pediatric dentists use it in their clinical practices.[13,14]

10. Trends followed in other disciplines. Great Britain began using N_2O in emergency medicine and for labor and delivery.[15] Podiatry first cited its use in the literature in 1966.[16] Many other health professions have begun using N_2O/O_2 sedation as a treatment modality for procedures not requiring general anesthesia.

11. Market predictions show an increase in the consumption of N_2O in the future.[17] The popularity of N_2O has waxed and waned over the years; however, it has remained in continuous use longer than any other drug. In spite of the advent of other attractive agents, N_2O has never been replaced.

REFERENCES

1. Smith WDA: *Under the influence: a history of nitrous oxide and oxygen anaesthesia,* London, 1982, Macmillan.
2. Langa H: *Relative analgesia in dental practice: inhalation analgesia with nitrous oxide,* Philadelphia, 1968, WB Saunders.
3. Fenster JM: How nobody invented anesthesia, *American Heritage of Invention & Technology* 12(1):24, 1996.
4. Jacobsohn PH: Dentistry's answer to "the humiliating spectacle": Dr. Wells and his discovery, *J Am Dent Assoc* 125:1576, 1994.
5. Menczer LF, Mittleman M, Wildsmith JA: Horace Wells, *J Am Dent Assoc* 110:773, 1985.
6. Chancellor JW: Dr. Wells' impact on dentistry and medicine, *J Am Dent Assoc* 125:1585, 1994.
7. Kennedy SK, Longnecker DE: History and principles of anesthesiology. In Hardman JG, Limbird LE, editors: *Goodman and Gillman's: the pharmacologic basis for therapeutics,* New York, 1996, McGraw-Hill.
8. Jacobsohn PH: What others said about Wells, *J Am Dent Assoc* 125:1583, 1994.
9. Jacobsohn PH: Remembering Dr. Menszer, *J Am Dent Assoc* 125:1582, 1994.
10. Rosenberg M: Personal communication with 2001 Horace Wells Club Award of Merit winner, October 2002.
11. MacAfee KA: Nitrous oxide. I. Historical perspective and patient selection, *Compend Contin Educ Dent* 10:352, 1989.
12. Malamed SF: Local anesthetics: dentistry's most important drugs, *J Am Dent Assoc* 125:1571, 1994.
13. ADA Survey Center: 1994 quarterly survey of dental practice, 3rd quarter, *ADA News,* 1994.
14. Davis MJ: Conscious sedation practices in pediatric dentistry: a survey of members of the American Board of Pediatric Dentistry College of Diplomates, *Pediatr Dent* 10:328, 1988.
15. Baskett PJF, Bennett JA: Pain relief in hospital: the more widespread use of nitrous oxide, *Br Med J* 2:509, 1971.
16. Arancia L: Nitrous oxide inhalation analgesia in ambulatory foot surgery, *J Am Coll Foot Surg* 5:111, 1966.
17. Frost & Sullivan, Inc: Anesthesia, gas monitoring markets to grow slightly, top $600 million by 2000, *Anesth Prog* 41:64, 1994.

3

Pain and Anxiety Management

Each year in the United States, 155 million people are in acute pain at least once[1] and pain is the primary complaint of approximately one half of the total number of persons seeking medical care.[1] Statistics also show that as many as 35 million people in the United States avoid the dental office because of their fear.[2] Fear and pain are interrelated. People will endure severe pain before seeking professional care often because of the fear that is associated with pain.[3] Individuals may find themselves in an emergency situation facing significant problems as a result of not having sought treatment at an earlier time when treatment could have increased the possibility of a favorable outcome.

Managing a patient's pain and anxiety before performing a medical procedure provides an optimal environment with benefits to both patient and clinician. Obviously, if you, the clinician, know that your patient is relaxed and comfortable, you can provide better service with less stress (Figure 3-1). There are many options currently available for pain and anxiety relief. Some options in certain situations will prove more advantageous than others. But for many procedures, several methods could be used. In those cases in which assistance in analgesia and anxiolysis would be beneficial, inhalation sedation using N_2O/O_2 should be a primary consideration.

I. Mechanism of Pain

A. Definition
1. As defined by the International Association for the Study of Pain, "pain is an unpleasant sensory and emotional experience arising from actual or potential tissue damage. The experience includes the perception of an uncomfortable stimulus and the response to that perception."[1]
B. Principles of action
1. The objective of pain is to provide damage protection to tissue by alerting the central nervous system (CNS) before or during a potentially damaging occurrence.
   a. Pain receptors (nociceptors) are the first to receive a stimulus. These receptors are nonspecialized, bare nerve endings that record the occurrence, intensity, duration, and location of the sensation.[4]
2. The theory of pain modulation suggests that impulses are altered along the way by an endogenous opioid system[5] (Figure 3-2).

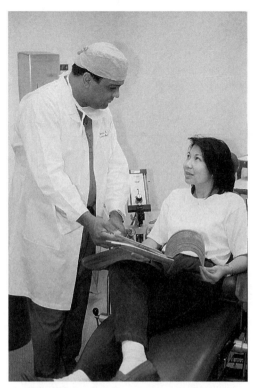

Figure 3-1   Reassuring an anxious patient.

3. Exogenous morphine binds to an opiate receptor, which accounts for its analgesic properties. Morphine is the drug to which endogenous opiates and other opioid drugs are compared.[5]
4. Research has attempted to determine the role of N_2O on the endogenous opioid system. Gillman[6] proposes that analgesic concentrations of N_2O may act directly on the opioid receptor and/or activate the release of endogenous opiates.
5. There is a physiobiochemical relationship between N_2O and opioids. Naloxone hydrochloride (Narcan) reverses the effects of opioid drugs and also has reversal action on N_2O and ketamine. This drug is most commonly used in acute opioid overdose situations.[7]
6. Endogenous endorphins, enkephalins, and dynorphins have been discovered as substances that bind to the opiate receptors, resulting in pain modulation.[4,5] Activation of the endogenous opioid system can be accomplished by pain and/or stress.[8] Research of the endogenous opioid system continues.
7. Reactions to pain vary from individual to individual and can vary from day to day. Many factors can influence pain reactions. Examples of these factors may be categorized as physical, mental, biochemical, psychologic, social, physiologic, cultural, and emotional.[1]

Trauma

Antagonism of endogenous analgesic substances and of inflammatory response (local anesthetics, NSAIDs, opioids, glucocorticoids, etc)

Pain

Nasal hood

Opioid receptors

Possible site of nitrous oxide receptors

Systemic opioids

Combination therapy "Balanced analgesia" "Multi-modal pain therapy"

Peripheral nerve

Central neural blockade (epidural/intrathecal local anesthetics, opioids, α_2-agonists)

Figure 3-2   Site of action of various analgesics.

C. Assessing and measuring pain
   1. There are a variety of scales intended to objectify the levels of pain to allow clinicians to act appropriately and alleviate discomfort. In many cases the scales have been helpful; however, some have not been useful. [9-11]
   2. A common scale depicts pain from 1 (very mild) to 5 (unbearable). Several other measures have been used; versions of various scales depict a range of facial images from comfortable to painful (Figure 3-3) for visually oriented populations such as children. Numeric scales prove useful when treating chronic pain because they can serve as baseline references over time.

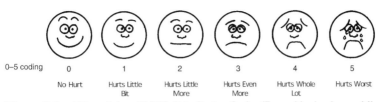

0–5 coding	0	1	2	3	4	5
	No Hurt	Hurts Little Bit	Hurts Little More	Hurts Even More	Hurts Whole Lot	Hurts Worst

Figure 3-3   Wong-Baker FACES Pain Rating Scale. (From Hockenberry MJ: *Wong's nursing care of infants and children*, ed 7, St Louis, 2003, Mosby.)

3. Even the simplest attempt to convey understanding of a patient's pain is appreciated. For example, try using a word for pain from the patient's native language. Some examples are listed in Box 3-1.
4. Asking patients about the extent of their pain communicates empathy toward the individuals. Problems occur when healthcare professionals are presumptuous about how a patient should or should not feel.
5. Healthcare professionals rely on a variety of continuing education and clinical experiences to guide them toward successful management of pain. Inherent in this process is the ability to adapt and change to specific patient complaints. This process is dynamic and continuous; each experience should develop better decision-making skills for the future. Healthcare professionals gain confidence with successful decisions, which ultimately benefit the patient.

II. Understanding Fear and Anxiety

A. Definitions

1. Anxiety: "A nonspecific feeling of apprehension, worry, uneasiness, or dread, the source of which may be vague or unknown. A normal

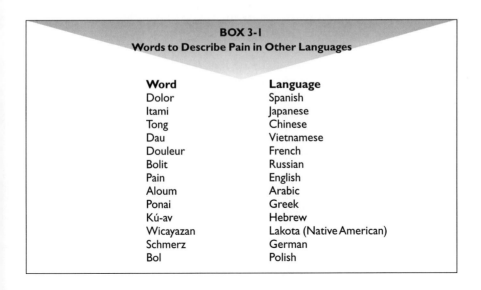

BOX 3-1
Words to Describe Pain in Other Languages

Word	Language
Dolor	Spanish
Itami	Japanese
Tong	Chinese
Dau	Vietnamese
Douleur	French
Bolit	Russian
Pain	English
Aloum	Arabic
Ponai	Greek
Kú-av	Hebrew
Wicayazan	Lakota (Native American)
Schmerz	German
Bol	Polish

reaction when one's body, lifestyle, values, or loved ones are threatened."[1]

2. Fear: "A feeling of fright or dread related to an identifiable source recognized by the individual."[1]

3. Phobia: "Any persistent and irrational fear of something specific, such as an object, activity, or situation that results in avoidance or desire to avoid the feared stimulus."[1]

B. Interaction between fear and pain

1. Fear and pain are so interrelated that they are often hard to separate. Both have physiologic and emotional components.[12] As pain increases, anxiety is heightened; as anxiety increases, pain becomes enhanced and therefore less tolerable.[4] In a medical setting, children cite fear of pain to be a significant obstacle.[13] When fear or pain is an issue, both must ultimately be managed.

C. Assessing and measuring fear and anxiety

1. Objectively quantifying a patient's fear or anxiety poses a dilemma similar to pain. There are several methods of assessing fear. Physiologic and behavioral signs often are overt indicators of fear ("white knuckle syndrome" is depicted in Figure 3-4). A simple interview with a patient will uncover otherwise unspoken concerns. Similar to scales used with pain, there are many measurement devices that indicate fear and anxiety. The literature overflows with suggested indicators.[14-16] Crying, clinging, sweating, syncope, refusal to cooperate, and obsessive talking may be interpreted as signs of fear. Chronic tardiness or last-minute appointment cancellations may also possibly be anxiety related.

2. Repeatedly, we hear of patients carrying fear into their adult lives precipitating from a negative childhood experience in a medical or dental setting. Often patients have preconceived expectations of pain stemming from attitudes and behaviors displayed by parents, siblings, co-workers, significant others, etc.[13] For those patients who have significant fear or phobias, referral to an appropriate professional (i.e., child psychologist, etc.) is suggested. There are many management options available for these individuals.[17] It is crucial that every effort be made to ensure a positive experience for each patient, child, or adult.

D. Acknowledgment of fear and anxiety

1. Good communication skills are necessary to facilitate the interpersonal interaction between the patient and provider. The basic fundamentals of good communication include warmth, empathy, and respect.[18] Empathy, which is best expressed through eye contact, has been cited as the greatest attribute a healthcare professional can possess.[19] By disclosing a genuine caring attitude, kindness, and concern for patients, healthcare providers can facilitate an interaction that allows for effective problem solving.[18] Patients do not care what professionals know until they know that these providers care.

2. Appropriate acknowledgment of patients' anxiety can solidify their confidence and allow an informed review of potential management options specific to every individual.[3]

Figure 3-4   Fear can be visible.

III. Sedation Levels as Defined by the ASA Practice Guidelines for Sedation and Analgesia by Non-Anesthesiologists[20](Box 3-2)

A. Definitions
1. Minimal sedation (anxiolysis): a drug-induced state during which patients respond normally to verbal commands. Although cognitive function and coordination may be impaired, ventilatory and cardiovascular functions are unaffected. When administering N_2O, minimal sedation is accomplished when concentrations are less than 50%.

BOX 3-2
ASA Continuum of Depth of Sedation

Minimal sedation (anxiolysis)
Moderate sedation-analgesia
Deep sedation-analgesia
General anesthesia

2. Moderate sedation-analgesia: a drug-induced depression of consciousness during which patients respond purposefully to verbal commands, either alone or accompanied by light tactile stimulation. No interventions are required to maintain a patent airway, and spontaneous ventilation is adequate. Cardiovascular function is usually maintained. Moderate sedation is achieved when N_2O concentrations are greater than 50%.

3. Deep sedation-analgesia: a drug-induced depression of consciousness during which patients cannot be easily aroused but respond purposefully following repeated or painful stimulation. The ability to independently maintain ventilatory function may be impaired. Patients may require assistance in maintaining a patent airway, and spontaneous ventilation may be inadequate. Cardiovascular function is usually maintained.

4. General anesthesia: a drug-induced loss of consciousness during which patients are not arousable, even by painful stimulation. The ability to independently maintain ventilatory function is often impaired. Patients often require assistance in maintaining a patent airway, and positive pressure ventilation may be required because of depressed spontaneous ventilation or drug-induced depression of neuromuscular function. Cardiovascular function may be impaired. With N_2O/O_2 it is difficult to reach the appropriate plane for performing a surgical procedure; however, although difficult it is possible to render a patient unconscious using N_2O/O_2.

B. Because sedation is a continuum, it is not always possible to predict how an individual patient will respond. Hence, practitioners intending to produce a given level of sedation should be able to rescue patients whose level of sedation becomes deeper than initially intended. Individuals administering moderate sedation-analgesia should be able to rescue patients who enter a state of deep sedation-analgesia, and those administering deep sedation-analgesia should be able to rescue patients who enter a state of general anesthesia.

IV. Spectrum of Pain and Anxiety Management Options

A. Several options are available for managing a patient's pain and anxiety. The spectrum begins with no intervention and ends with general anesthesia (Figure 3-5). There are methods that use pharmacologic agents and others that do not. Options for consideration will be discussed briefly. For additional information regarding any of these, several reputable texts and other resources are available.[3]

1. Noninvasive, nonpharmacologic approach to sedation
   a. Iatrosedation may be defined as words and actions used by a clinician to facilitate a trusting relationship and positive rapport with a patient. This conscious choice of verbal and nonverbal communication is a vital component of every patient-operator interaction.[21] Positive attitudes, welcoming smiles, and a genuine display of kindness and con-

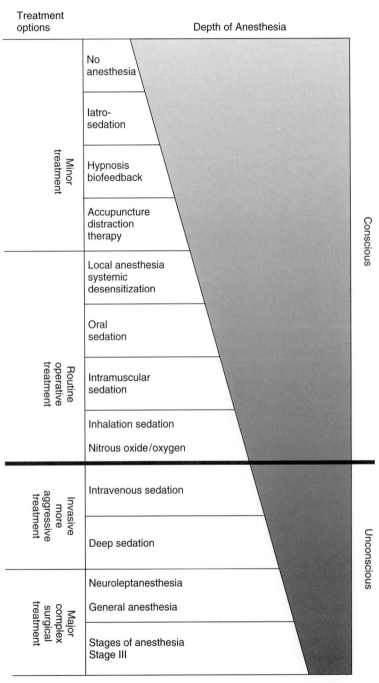

Figure 3-5 Pain and anxiety management options.

cern reassure patients and may be all that is necessary to allay fear and anxiety. Language and actions are calm, slow, relaxing, and gentle.[22] Most often iatrosedation is used to facilitate the effectiveness of pharmacologic modalities.

b. Hypnosis is another nonpharmacologic method of providing pain and anxiety relief. Promoters suggest that hypnosis makes use of an individual's natural abilities.[23] Further study and training are necessary before using these techniques in addition to patient preparation. Not everyone is hypnosuggestable; therefore this option is not reliable for all patients.

c. Acupuncture and acupressure are similar to hypnosis because they require further education and training before they are used.[24] Their disadvantage, similar to hypnosis, is unreliability for every patient.

d. Systematic desensitization, relaxation therapy, biofeedback, distraction, and other coping strategies may be used to manage patient fear and anxiety. With the exception of distraction, these methods usually require the assistance of specialized professionals. Many resources are available that provide such services and/or information. Distraction mechanisms are intended to divert the individual's attention away from a fear-provoking stimulus. Examples of such distractions are reading materials in reception areas, music via office speakers or headphones, television, movies, aromatherapy, virtual reality headsets, and even manicures during dental procedures!

e. Transcutaneous electrical nerve stimulation (TENS) and electronic dental anesthesia (EDA) are pain-relieving methods that use electricity to prevent impulses from reaching the brain. Large A-fibers are stimulated electrically until the patient signals a tolerable twitching sensation. According to the Melzack and Wall[25] gate theory, impulses will not be propagated further, thus reducing pain. TENS also acts with the endogenous opioid system to produce endorphins and enkephalins.[26] Historically TENS has been used in physical therapy; however, dentistry has given TENS and EDA more exposure. The first and only blind, controlled study of TENS effectiveness was done by Clark.[27] Several other studies indicate significant analgesic effects.[28-30]

2. Invasive, pharmacologic approach to sedation

a. Conscious patients

i. Local anesthesia is described as a loss of sensation in a localized area caused by an anesthetic agent that blocks the neurotransmission of impulses to the brain. The injection is known to be a primary source of the fear and anxiety that providers continuously attempt to manage.[31]

ii. The oral route may be used to administer pharmacologic agents for the purpose of relaxing an apprehensive individual without producing unconsciousness.[3] Administering drugs orally is universally accepted by the general population. Patient cooperation is necessary but usually not problematic, except with children in some cases. Oral medication has a latent period of 30 minutes, peaking at approximately 1 hour, and may be considerably affected by gastric contents. Duration of action and recovery are prolonged, and an escort is often required. There is no mechanism for titration with oral medication.

iii. The intramuscular (IM) route of administration is accomplished by direct injection into muscular tissue. Clinical action is more rapid than with the oral route, and absorption is more reliable. Disadvantages are the inability to titrate the drug, prolonged duration, incomplete recovery, and the necessity of an injection.[3]

iv. The inhalation route of administration of medication offers many advantages and few disadvantages. The clinical effect is rapid, titration is possible, and elimination of the drug is usually rapid. This will be discussed as it pertains to N_2O in greater detail in Chapter 4.

v. The IV route of administration is the direct deposition of drug into the circulatory system. This allows for very rapid response and onset of action. It is titratable and therefore can be tailored for a specific procedure. Recovery time can be prolonged and the patient requires an escort[3] (Figure 3-6).

b. Unconscious patients

i. General anesthesia has been used extensively in the health professions since the discovery of N_2O and ether as anesthetics. Patient cooperation is not a factor for its effectiveness, which is often the reason why this modality is selected. Patients who are unmanageable for any reason are potential candidates for general anesthesia. To perform this technique the practitioner must complete additional educational requirements and assume greater liability.[3]

Figure 3-6   IV sedation.

B. Whichever option is chosen, careful and competent decision-making skills are vital. Select the management option that best suits the situation at hand. Because each person responds differently to nonpharmacologic and pharmacologic methods of treatment, remember that an individual's responses are variable on any given day. Psychologic and physiologic factors must be considered at each meeting with the patient. When one modality is insufficient or undesirable, another may prove effective.

REFERENCES

 1. Thomas CL, editor: *Taber's cyclopedic medical dictionary,* Philadelphia, 1997, FA Davis.
 2. Consensus Conference: Anesthesia and sedation in the dental office, *J Am Med Assoc* 254:1073, 1985.
 3. Malamed SF: *Sedation: a guide to patient management,* ed 4, St Louis, 2003, Mosby.
 4. Stoelting RK: *Pharmacology and physiology in anesthetic practice,* ed 2, Philadelphia, 1991, JB Lippincott.
 5. Hirst M: The changing nature of pain control: clinical aspects of endorphins and enkephalins, *J Canadian Dent Assoc* 51:493, 1985.
 6. Gillman MA: Analgesic (subanesthetic) nitrous oxide interacts with the endogenous opioid system: a review of the evidence, *Life Sciences* 39:1209, 1986.
 7. Reisine T, Pasternak G: Opioid analgesics and antagonists. In Hardman JG, Limbird LE, editors: *Goodman and Gillman's: the pharmacologic basis of therapeutics,* ed 9, New York, 1996, McGraw-Hill.
 8. Hargreaves KM, Dubner R: Mechanisms of pain and analgesia. In Dionne RA, Phero JC, editors: *Management of pain and anxiety in dental practice,* New York, 1991, Elsevier Science Publishing.
 9. Kohr J: Measuring your patient's pain, *RN* 58:39, 1995.
10. Gujol MC: A survey of pain assessment and management practices among critical care nurses, *Am J Crit Care* 3:123, 1994.
11. McCafery M, Richey KJ: Techniques of pain assessment, *Nurse Week* 5:16, 1992.
12. Pawlicki RE: Psychological/behavior techniques in managing pain and anxiety in the dental patient. In Dionne RA, Phero JC, editors: *Management of pain and anxiety in dental practice,* New York, 1991, Elsevier Science Publishing.
13. Prins PJ: Anxiety in medical settings. In Ollendick TH, King NJ, Yule W, editors: *International handbook of phobic and anxiety disorders in children and adolescents,* New York, 1994, Plenum Press.
14. Mendola P, O'Shea RM, Zielezny MA: Validity and reliability of the interval scale of anxiety response, *Anesth Prog* 34:202, 1987.
15. Parkin SF: The assessment of two dental anxiety rating scales for children, *J Dent Child* 55:269, 1988.
16. Elter JR, Strauss RP, Beck JD: Assessing dental anxiety, dental care use and oral status in older adults, *J Am Dent Assoc* 128:591, 1997.
17. Weinstein P, Nathan JE: The challenge of fearful and phobic children, *Dent Clin North Am* 32:667, 1988.
18. Doebling S, Rowe MM: Negative perceptions of dental stimuli and their effects on dental fear, *J Dent Hygiene* 74:110, 2000.
19. Ketchum C: Freedom from fear, *RDH* 3:14, 1995.
20. ASA Task Force: Practice guidelines for sedation and analgesia by non-anesthesiologists, *Anesthesiology* 96(4):1007, 2002.
21. Stracher K: The role of suggestion in conscious-sedation, *Anesth Prog* 23:59, 1976.

22. Ross ID: Fear control with nitrous oxide sedation, *SAAD Digest* 9:69, 1992.
23. Simpson MA et al: *Hypnosis in dentistry: a handbook for clinical use*, Springfield, Ill, 1985, Charles C Thomas.
24. Santamaria LB: Non-pharmacologic techniques for treatment of post-operative pain, *Minerva Anestesiol* 56:359, 1990.
25. Melzack R, Wall P: Pain mechanisms: a new theory, *Science* 150:971, 1965.
26. Malamed SF: *Handbook of local anesthesia*, ed 4, St Louis, 1997, Mosby.
27. Clark MS et al: An evaluation of the clinical analgesia/anesthesia efficacy on acute pain using the high frequency neural modulator in various dental settings, *Oral Surg* 63:501, 1987.
28. Christensen GJ: Electronic anesthesia: research and thoughts, *J Calif Dent Assoc* 15:46, 1987.
29. Hochman R: Neurotransmitter modulator (TENS) for control of dental operative pain, *J Am Dent Assoc* 116:208, 1988.
30. Malamed SF et al: Electronic dental anesthesia for restorative dentistry, *Anesth Prog* 36:195, 1989.
31. Milgrom P et al: Four dimensions of fear of dental injections, *J Am Dent Assoc* 128:756, 1997.

SUGGESTED READINGS

Heitkemper T, Layne C, Sullivan DM: Brief treatment of children's dental pain and anxiety, *Percept Mot Skills* 76:192, 1993.

Kaufman E, Jastak JT: Sedation for outpatient dental procedures, *Compend Dent* 16:462, 1995.

Nathan JE: Management of the difficult child: a survey of pediatric dentists' use of restraints, sedation and general anesthesia, *J Dent Child* 56(4):293, 1989.

Slavin HC: What we know about pain, *J Am Dent Assoc* 127:1536, 1996.

4

Comparison of N_2O/O_2 Sedation to Other Sedation Methods

N_2O/O_2 sedation has many advantages over other pain and anxiety management options. There are many indications for its use and the disadvantages are few; for these reasons it can be a useful sedative method. The majority of these advantages deal with the pharmacokinetics of the drug itself (Box 4-1). Judge for yourself how the N_2O/O_2 option compares with others.

I. Comparative Analysis of N_2O/O_2 Therapy with Other Methods

A. Analgesic properties (pain control)
   1. Chapman, Arrowood, and Beecher[1] state that a mixture of 20% N_2O and 80% O_2 has the same analgesic equipotence as 15 mg of morphine. Other methods verifying the analgesic efficacy of N_2O have been reported.[2]
   2. The level of pain control afforded by N_2O can vary from patient to patient because of individual biovariability; however, the analgesic properties of N_2O are well recognized and its potency is significant.[1] These analgesic properties are useful even with the severe pain associated with myocardial infarction.[3] N_2O has the ability to raise the patient's pain threshold when administered before intraoral injections in dentistry.[4]
   3. N_2O/O_2 is also advantageous when other analgesic drugs are contraindicated (i.e., allergy).
   4. Fear affects an individual's ability to tolerate pain; painful stimuli can be exaggerated in an anxious patient. A common fear is fear of an injection or a needle (i.e., vaccination), which can intensify an individual's reaction to pain.[5] N_2O has the ability to manage both pain and fear.
B. Anxiolytic properties (sedative effects)
   1. Patient anxiety has long been associated with oral healthcare.[6] A person's mental ability to cope with certain situations can depend on such things as age, sex, previous experiences, and personality characteristics.[7]
   2. N_2O/O_2 therapy can significantly assist patients in handling their fear or anxiety by producing sedation or a sense of well-being. Sedation enables

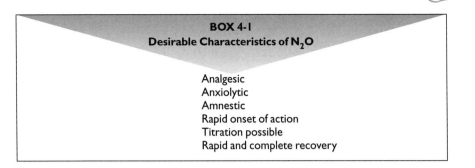

BOX 4-1
Desirable Characteristics of N_2O

Analgesic
Anxiolytic
Amnestic
Rapid onset of action
Titration possible
Rapid and complete recovery

the patient to become calm, relaxed, and able to tolerate the situation better or with no difficulty.

   a. This relaxed feeling has a positive effect on the patient's pain threshold.
   b. Mood changes with N_2O have been studied. Zacny et al[8] report positive mood changes in patients with high anxiety and in those with low anxiety.
   c. Patients with dental fear were treated with N_2O sedation. Results were favorable; this study reassessed patients 1 year later. The results showed that the N_2O treatment method still had a positive effect.[9]
3. In treatment of pediatric patients, N_2O/O_2 has been shown to facilitate positive behavior and lowered anxiety levels on sequential visits.[10] It is a continuing goal of all healthcare professionals to prevent negative early childhood experiences to reduce the number of fearful adults. Ultimately, the goal is to provide patients with enough positive experiences that they do not require N_2O/O_2 sedation in the future.

C. Amnestic properties
1. The amnestic property of N_2O/O_2 sedation is another of its positive attributes.[11] Postoperatively, patients often state they cannot recall the severity of their pain or anxiety nor its duration.
2. The passage of time tends to become unclear under N_2O/O_2 sedation. A patient may remark how quickly time passed during a time-intensive procedure.[4]

D. Onset of action
1. N_2O/O_2 sedation has a rapid onset of action. Because of the pharmacologic characteristics of N_2O, clinical effects may begin in less than 30 seconds, with peak effects occurring in less than 5 minutes.
2. Another conscious-sedative modality that closely parallels the rapid onset of clinical action of N_2O/O_2 is IV sedation.

E. Titration
1. Titration is the process of administering a drug incrementally to a specific level or endpoint of sedation. It allows for the exact amount of the drug necessary to be delivered to every patient at every appointment. Titration is very easily accomplished with N_2O/O_2

sedation. N_2O is one of several drugs that accommodate the concept of titration well.

    2. Titration is possible with IV sedation; however, in this case the drug cannot quickly or easily be decreased or eliminated.

F. Recovery

    1. Inhalation of N_2O/O_2 allows for complete recovery using 100% pure oxygen for a minimum of 5 minutes after termination of the drug. Depending upon patient assessment, individual recovery time may vary. Recovery will be discussed further in Chapter 14.

G. Acceptance

    1. Patient acceptance of the procedure has been well documented. Berge[12] states that the acceptance rate is the same for oral surgery procedures as it is for general dentistry.

II. Combining N_2O/O_2 Sedation with Other Methods

A. N_2O/O_2 sedation is enhanced with sophrology, the science of the spoken word. Soothing, calm, humorous, encouraging words and actions of the operator facilitate the relaxing effects of the drug.[4,13] Investigators believe the psychologic preparation of the patient before N_2O/O_2 administration has a significant impact on its effects.[14-16]

B. Weinstein and Nathan[17] indicate that N_2O used in combination with distraction techniques was more effective than distraction with a placebo gas when working with children. They also suggest that the combination of N_2O/O_2 and hypnosis and imagery was effective with their population.[17]

Figure 4-1   Music and N_2O/O_2 sedation (2003). (Courtesy Dr. Elizabeth Barr, Denver, Colorado.)

C. Another combination cited as effective with pediatric patients is the use of audioanalgesia and N_2O/O_2. The addition of music as an adjuvant to N_2O/O_2 sedation was positive for the children studied (Figure 4-1).[18] Music has been used as a method for calming, relaxing, and distracting individuals in the healthcare setting since the era of unusually loud music used for distraction (also known as "white sound") in the late 1950s and early 1960s.[19,20]

D. Quarnstrom[21] was more successful in his research when he combined N_2O/O_2 and EDA, compared with using each modality alone.

E. Oral premedication may be used safely with N_2O/O_2 sedation.[22] Diazepam and meperidine have been cited as drugs used concomitantly with N_2O.

F. The combination that deserves special attention is that of N_2O/O_2 and local anesthesia. The benefits of local anesthesia are apparent; N_2O/O_2 should not be used as a substitute for local anesthesia but rather as an adjuvant to it. If N_2O/O_2 is administered alone in a situation that also requires local anesthesia, the patient may blame the N_2O/O_2 unfairly for not eliminating the pain. The patient will be less likely to trust N_2O/O_2 in the future. Local anesthesia and N_2O/O_2 combined offer a superior pain and anxiety management option.

REFERENCES

1. Chapman WP, Arrowood JG, Beecher HK: The analgesic effects of low concentrations of nitrous oxide compared in man with morphine sulphate, *J Clin Invest* 22:871, 1943.

2. Pirec V, Patterson TH, Thapar P: Effects of subanesthetic concentrations of nitrous oxide on cold-pressor pain in humans, *Pharm Biochem Behav* 51:323, 1995.

3. Thompson PL, Lown B: Nitrous oxide as an analgesic in acute myocardial infarction, *JAMA* 235:924, 1976.

4. Malamed SF: *Sedation: a guide to patient management*, ed 4, St Louis, 2003, Mosby.

5. Murray JB: Psychology of the pain experience. In Weisenberg M, editor: *Pain: clinical and experimental perspectives*, St Louis, 1975, Mosby.

6. Doebling S, Rowe MM: Negative perceptions of dental stimuli and their effects on dental fear, *JDH* 74(II):110, 2000.

7. Doerr PA et al: Factors associated with dental anxiety, *J Am Dent Assoc* 129:1111, 1998.

8. Zacny JP et al: Preoperative dental anxiety and mood changes during nitrous oxide inhalation, *J Am Dent Assoc* 133:82, 2002.

9. Willumsen T et al: One-year follow-up of patients treated for dental fear: effects of cognitive therapy, applied relaxations, and nitrous oxide sedation, *Acta Odontol Scand* 59(6):335, 2001.

10. Veerkamp JS et al: Anxiety reduction with nitrous oxide: a permanent solution? *J Dent Child* 62:44, 1995.

11. Ramsey DS, Leonesio RJ, Whitney CW et al: Paradoxical effects of nitrous oxide on human memory, *Psychopharmacology* 106:370, 1992.

12. Berge TI: Acceptance and side effects of nitrous oxide oxygen sedation for oral surgical procedures, *Acta Odontol Scand* 57(4):201, 1999.

13. Winland RD: Humor: part of the treatment plan, *Gen Dentistry* 45(5):414, 1997.

14. Patel B et al: The use of hypnosis in dentistry: a review, *Dent Update* 27(4):198, 2002.

15. Dworkin SF et al: Analgesic effects of nitrous oxide with controlled painful stimuli, *JADA* 107:581, 1983.

16. Chaves JF: Recent advances in the application of hypnosis to pain management, *Am J Clin Hypn* 37:117, 1994.
17. Weinstein P, Nathan JE: The challenge of fearful and phobic children, *Dent Clin North Am* 32:667, 1988.
18. Anderson WD: The effectiveness of audio-nitrous oxide-oxygen psychosedation on dental behavior of a child, *J Pedodontics* 5:3, 1980.
19. Gardner, Licklider: Auditory analgesia in dental operation, *J Am Dent Assoc* 59:1144, 1959.
20. Robson, Davenport: The effects of white sound and music upon superficial pain threshold, *Can J Anaesth* 9:105, 1962.
21. Quarnstrom FC: Clinical experience with TENS and TENS combined with nitrous oxide-oxygen, *Anesth Prog* 36:66, 1989.
22. Jastak JT, Paravecchio R: An analysis of 1331 sedations using inhalation, intravenous, or other techniques, *J Am Dent Assoc* 91:1242, 1975.

5

Physical Properties and Pharmacokinetics of N₂O

The conscientious healthcare provider offering N_2O/O_2 sedation to patients must be knowledgeable about the actions of the drug. N_2O has many favorable attributes. Several of these characteristics relate to the pharmacologic properties of the drug and some are particularly advantageous when using N_2O for general anesthesia; however, the same principles also prove noteworthy in the ambulatory setting. Although there may be disagreement about whether N_2O deserves the "ideal" label, many agree that its role in healthcare is fundamental.

I. Physical and Chemical Properties of N₂O

A. Dinitrogen monoxide (N_2O) is a stable, linear compound that is chemically diagrammed as
N≡N=O. It is a sweet-smelling, colorless gas.

B. The boiling point of N_2O, which is 88.5° C (127° F), indicates that it is a gas at room temperature. When compressed into a cylinder, N_2O becomes a liquid.

C. The substance itself is nonflammable; however, N_2O supports combustion. If the gas comes in contact with a combustible substance or flame of 1200° F, decomposition of the gas will occur. If the decomposition occurs at high temperature and elevated pressure (inside a cylinder or high-pressure pipeline), a violent chemical reaction such as an explosion will occur. If N_2O is present near an open flame, the flame will burn brighter.[1]

D. *Because N_2O like O_2 is an oxidizing gas, no hydrocarbon compounds such as lubricants, grease, or oil should be used on any N_2O storage, distribution, or dispensing equipment.* Of further concern is the operation of such equipment in a manner that increases the temperature of the N_2O. The most common example is the quick opening of valves, which causes a rapid pressure increase. The phenomenon known as the *heat of compression* can increase the temperature of the gas and metal to a level that ignites any hydrocarbon contaminants and causes a chemical reaction resulting in fire or explosion. This reaction can occur with any organic contaminant acting as a fuel.

E. The molecular weight of N_2O is 44. Its specific gravity is 1.53, which indicates that it is heavier than air (gr = 1) or pure O_2 (gr = 1.1).

F. N_2O is found in minimal concentrations (6 ppm) in the atmosphere.[2] Anesthetic N_2O contributes approximately 1% of that total amount.[3] As ultraviolet (UV) light combines with N_2O and O_2, free radicals (i.e., nitric oxide) are produced, which can affect the ozone.[4] Several natural and man-made methods release N_2O into the atmosphere (e.g., burning of pine wood). Recent literature suggests that N_2O enters the environment via rivers, denitrification of soil, and plants and trees.[5-7] This naturally-occurring product has minimal effect when compared to other gases (e.g., carbon dioxide, water, and methane) on global warming and contributes approximately 4% to the "greenhouse effect."[8]

II. Physical and Chemical Properties of O_2

A. Discovery
   1. Many early scientists such as Bayen, Borch, and Scheele prepared O_2 but did not recognize the significance of their findings.[9]
   2. Joseph Priestley in England was credited with discovering not only N_2O but O_2, carbon monoxide, sulfur dioxide, and ammonia. Priestley, a British chemist, is considered one of the founders of modern chemistry because of his contributions to the field of science.[10]
B. Preparation
   1. O_2 is primarily prepared by fractional evaporation of liquid air or by heating potassium chlorate using manganese dioxide as a catalyst. Air separation plants make 99% of the gas. O_2 costs approximately 5 cents per cubic foot for small quantities.[9]
   2. Air is cooled and compressed until it liquefies. O_2 compresses to a pale blue liquid at $-183°$ C and is strongly paramagnetic.
   3. Nitrogen (N) and other elements evaporate, leaving liquid O_2.
C. Characteristics
   1. In a gaseous state O_2 is odorless, colorless, and tasteless.
   2. It makes up approximately 21% of the earth's atmosphere and makes up 49.2% of the earth's crust. The human body is 61% oxygen and 90% of water is oxygen. Oxygen is the third most abundant element in the sun and is thought to be part of its energy source.[9]
   3. The molecular weight of O_2 is 32; its specific gravity is 1.1 (air = 1) and its atomic weight is 15.9. The atomic weight of oxygen was used as the standard for comparison of other elements until carbon 12 replaced it as the standard in 1961.[9]
   4. Like N_2O, O_2 supports combustion but is not itself flammable. It reacts similarly to N_2O when it contacts a combustible material such as oils, grease, or flammable materials.
   5. O_2 is a compressed gas in cylinders. The dial in the regulator gauge accurately depicts the O_2 content in the cylinder. As the gas is consumed, the dial changes proportionally.
   6. Oxygen is highly reactive and combines with most elements. It is a component within hundreds of thousands of organic compounds.

D. Uses

1. There are many uses for O_2. The steel industry is one of the largest consumers of O_2. O_2 is also used for welding and lighting and as a propellant in rockets. It is widely used in the medical field for surgical procedures, treating anaerobic infections, and hypoxia. Commercially, O_2 consumption is estimated at 20 million short tons per year in the United States.[9]

2. O_2 is the required component of N_2O when N_2O is used for sedation. Current sedation equipment described guarantees a minimum O_2 delivery of 30%. This provides an amount of O_2 greater than that found naturally in atmospheric air, which is significant for patient safety during N_2O/O_2 administration. It is common to use approximately 2.5 tanks of O_2 to every 1 tank of N_2O during sedation procedures.

III. Pharmacokinetic Properties of N_2O

A. The pharmacokinetic aspects of a drug affect its uptake, distribution, metabolism, and elimination in the body. Inhaled agents such as N_2O express their actions on the body by moving across partial pressure gradients. The agent moves from a higher- to a lower-pressure gradient. Uptake, distribution, onset of action, and ultimately, recovery from anesthesia or sedation depend on the solubility and potency of the drug. The interaction between a drug, the brain, and other tissues until equilibrium is reached is expressed in values called *partition coefficients*. These values indicate the ease or difficulty of drug transfer to the brain and body.

1. The difference between the partial pressures of a gas (N_2O) and a liquid (blood) indicates how quickly the agent crosses the pulmonary membrane and enters the bloodstream. This is called the *blood-gas partition coefficient*. N_2O crosses the alveolar membrane easily. The solubility of the drug then determines how quickly equilibration occurs and clinical action begins.

   a. If a drug is highly soluble, it will diffuse immediately into the blood and be distributed throughout the body. Its blood-gas partition coefficient will be high, indicating that more drug and/or more time will be necessary to achieve equilibration or the level necessary for movement of the agent to the brain.

   b. If a drug is relatively insoluble, equilibrium will be achieved quickly. The blood-brain barrier will be crossed rapidly, allowing the drug to reach the brain. The onset of clinical action will then also be rapid.

   c. N_2O is an example of a relatively insoluble drug. Its blood-gas partition coefficient is 0.47. It remains unchanged in the blood and does not combine with any blood elements; the O_2 component is not available for use in the body because N_2O does not break down. Uptake by the body is limited, indicating that equilibrium is achieved quickly. Therefore, peak clinical effects may be seen within 3 to 5 minutes after initiation of the agent.

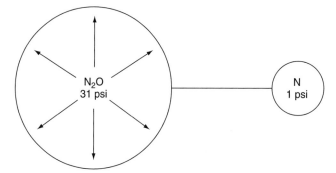

Figure 5-1 N_2O will diffuse from the blood into closed air-containing spaces in the body, especially an occluded middle ear. N_2O will continue to move into the space until equilibrium is achieved with the alveolar N_2O concentration. Because N_2O is 31 times more soluble in blood than N_2, more N_2O will diffuse into the occluded middle ear space than N_2 diffuses out. The higher the concentration of inspired N_2O, the more N_2O accumulates in the occluded middle ear, resulting in increased middle ear pressure and possibly diminished hearing postoperatively.

    d. There is a major difference in partial pressure gradients between N_2O and nitrogen (N_2). The partial pressure of N_2O is approximately 31 times greater than that of N_2 (Figure 5-1). Because of this, N_2O rapidly replaces the N_2 occupying any body space. Not only does N_2O physically replace N_2, but it also increases the volume and/or pressure of that space depending on its rigid or nonrigid confines. Specific conditions regarding this phenomenon are described in Chapter 9 (Figure 5-2).
  2. Other partition coefficients of N_2O between tissues, muscles, and fat are low. Equilibration occurs quickly in these instances because of the inability of the tissues to hold N_2O. Because of this, N_2O is not stored in the body to any extent; thus elimination is not impeded.[11]
B. Eger[12] introduced the concept of the concentration effect (Figure 5-3) of N_2O upon induction. The concentration effect occurs when high concentrations of N_2O are delivered to the patient (70% N_2O). These high concentrations are often delivered during general anesthesia.
  1. At high concentrations, alveolar partial pressures are reached rapidly and there is little decrease in the concentration of the gas. In addition, when delivering these high concentrations of N_2O, the volume of inspired gas is increased. Negative pressure is produced, drawing more gas into the lungs and increasing the volume.
  2. At lower concentrations the concentration effect is not significant. When administering analgesic percentages of N_2O, the rate of uptake is not as important.
C. As high concentrations of N_2O promote the rapid uptake of the gas, there is a simultaneous effect occurring with the other gases being administered. The rapid uptake of N_2O allows the second gas to be drawn in much faster than it would normally if it were being administered alone. This phenomenon, the second-gas effect (Figure 5-4), allows minimal amounts of a more potent anesthetic to be administered simultaneously with N_2O.[12]

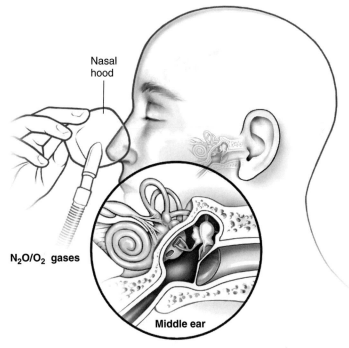

Nasal hood

N$_2$O/O$_2$ gases

Middle ear

Figure 5-2 Effects of gas solubility.

10 mph = 10% N$_2$O concentration

80 mph = 80% N$_2$O concentration with increased vacuum and increased gas uptake (Ethrane)

Figure 5-3 Concentration effect of N$_2$O.

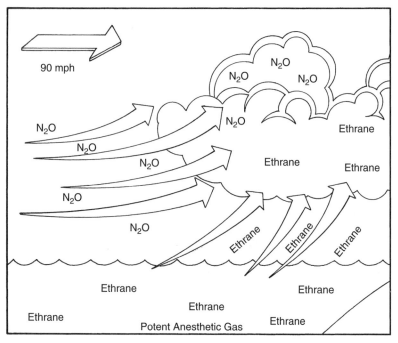

Figure 5-4   Second-gas effect associated with N_2O.

D. N_2O is not metabolized through the liver. Ninety-nine percent of it is elimi-nated through the lungs without significant biotransformation.[13] A minis-cule (0.004%) amount of N_2O is metabolized in the gastrointestinal tract. Reduction occurs by the anaerobic bacteria *Pseudomonas* and produces potentially toxic free radicals.[14,15] This process does not pose any significant threat to the body systems.

E. N_2O is difficult to use at extreme altitudes (i.e., above 10,000 feet). Because of the barometric pressure change, air ambulances and those administering N_2O/O_2 sedation at significant elevations must be aware of the need for an increase in N_2O concentration to obtain the same effects as at sea level.[13] In Denver, Colorado, United States (5280 feet elevation) for example, a 5% increase in N_2O may be necessary as compared with a location at sea level.

IV. Potency of Anesthetic Agents

A. The potency of an anesthetic agent indicates how strong or powerful the drug is or how effective it is at producing anesthesia. There are many drugs available for general anesthesia that vary widely in potency.

1. N_2O is the least potent (weakest) of all inhalation general anesthetics.

2. Drug potency is determined by assessing the minimum alveolar concentration (MAC). MAC is defined as the amount of drug necessary to prevent movement in 50% of subjects responding to surgical incision.[16]

3. The MAC for N$_2$O is 104% to 105%. This value indicates that at normal atmospheric pressure N$_2$O alone is not able to produce profound surgical anesthesia. N$_2$O can be used as the sole anesthetic agent under hyperbaric conditions.[17]

4. The MAC value and limited potency of N$_2$O add tremendously to its safety. Some anesthetic agents and their corresponding MAC values are listed in Box 5-1.

B. Halothane, isoflurane, enflurane, desflurane, and sevoflurane are examples of more potent inhalation agents used for general anesthesia. Although their benefits are many, they also possess several negative factors, including toxicity, biotransformation, solubility, and general complication issues sometimes resulting in negative effects on organ systems.

C. N$_2$O can be used in combination with more potent inhaled agents to decrease the percentage of inhaled agents required and possibly diminish unwanted toxic side effects, as well as to be more cost effective. The second-gas effect does not play a role per se in this regard. The second-gas effect is primarily relevant when trying to achieve equilibrium of the potent anesthetic agent such as at induction.

V. Toxicity

A. When N$_2$O is used on healthy patients for clinical procedures of reasonable length, toxicity is insignificant or nonexistent. The effects of N$_2$O on body systems are discussed in Chapter 9.

B. Research studies done with both animals and humans indicate that prolonged exposure to N$_2$O can have a negative effect on vitamin B$_{12}$ and its role in DNA synthesis. N$_2$O oxidizes the cobalt atom of vitamin B$_{12}$ thereby inactivating its dependent enzyme, methionine synthetase. This action results in bone marrow depression. Further discussion of the effects associated with prolonged N$_2$O exposure is found in Chapter 17.

BOX 5-1

Minimum Alveolar Concentration (MAC) Values for Inhalation Anesthetics

Anesthetic	MAC Value
Desflurane	4.6%
Enflurane	1.6%
Halothane	0.75%
Isoflurane	1.2%
Nitrous oxide	104%
Sevoflurane	1.7%

REFERENCES

1. Fettes WC: Personal communication, August 1996.
2. Maskell K, Mintzer IM, Callander BA: Basic science of climate change, *Lancet* 342:1027, 1993.
3. Sherman SJ, Cullen BF: Nitrous oxide and the greenhouse effect, *Anesthesiology* 68:816, 1988.
4. Dale O, Husum B: Nitrous oxide: a threat to personnel and global environment? *Acta Anaesthesiol Scand* 38:777, 1994.
5. Cole JJ, Caraco NF: Emissions of nitrous oxide from a tidal, freshwater river, the Hudson River, New York, *Environ Sci Technol* 35(6): 991, 2001.
6. Barton L, Schipper LA: Regulation of nitrous oxide emissions from soils irrigated with dairy farm effluent, *J Environ Quality* 30(6):1881, 2001.
7. Xu H et al: N_2O emission by trees under natural conditions, *Environ Sci* 22(5):7, 2001.
8. Dookun R, Lyne JP, Robb ND: Nitrous oxide: past, present and future, *SAAD Digest* 14(1-2):13, 1997.
9. Lide DR: *CRC handbook of chemistry and physics,* ed 81, New York, 2001, CRC Press.
10. Microsoft Encarta Online Encyclopedia: *Joseph Priestley,* http://encarta.msn.com, 2002.
11. Eger EI II: Pharmacokinetics. In Eger EI II, editor: *Nitrous oxide N_2O,* New York, 1985, Elsevier Science Publishing.
12. Eger EI II: Uptake and distribution. In Miller RD, editor: *Anesthesia,* ed 4, vol 1, New York, 1994, Churchill Livingstone.
13. Stoelting RD: *Pharmacology and physiology in anesthetic practice,* ed 2, Philadelphia, 1991, JB Lippincott.
14. Hong K et al: Metabolism of nitrous oxide by human and rat intestinal contents, *Anesthesiology* 52:16, 1980.
15. Hong K et al: Biotransformation of nitrous oxide, *Anesthesiology* 53:354, 1980.
16. Eger EI II, Saidman LJ, Brandstater B: Minimum alveolar anesthetic concentration: a standard of anesthetic potency, *Anesthesiology* 26:756, 1965.
17. Eger EI II: MAC. In Eger EI II, editor: *Nitrous oxide N_2O,* New York, 1985, Elsevier Science Publishing.

SUGGESTED READINGS

Cullen DJ: Anesthetic pharmacology and critical care, *Acute Care* 14-15:3, 1988-1989.
Dale O, Brown JR Jr: Clinical pharmacokinetics of the inhalational anaesthetics, *Clin Pharmacokinet* 12:145, 1987.
Hardman JG, Limbird LE, editors: *Goodman and Gillman's: the pharmacologic basis of therapeutics,* ed 9, New York, 1996, McGraw-Hill.
Joyce JL: Inhalation anesthetics, *AORN J* 52:77, 1990.
Longnecker DE, Miller FL: Pharmacology of inhalation anesthetics. In Rogers M et al, editors: *Principles and practice of anesthesiology,* St Louis, 1993, Mosby.
Stenqvist O: Nitrous oxide kinetics, *Acta Anaesthesiol Scand* 38:757, 1994.
Stoelting RD: *Pharmacology and physiology in anesthetic practice,* ed 2, Philadelphia, 1991, JB Lippincott.

6

Manufacturing and Distribution of N₂O and O₂ Gases

I. Manufacturing

A. Process and storage
  1. The manufacturing process for N_2O is relatively simple. The raw ingredient, ammonium nitrate (NH_4NO_3), is supplied as a clear liquid or as solid, pellet-sized particles. This material is used for fertilizer and as a primary ingredient of explosives. Unfortunately, it was used in the infamous bombing of the Alfred Murrah Federal Building in Oklahoma City in April 1994.
  2. To make N_2O, NH_4NO_3 is heated to approximately 250° C. At that point the NH_4NO_3 decomposes into N_2O, water (steam), and some contaminants ($NH_4NO_3 \rightarrow N_2O + 2\ H_2O$). The gas mixture is cooled to ambient temperature, the steam is condensed, and the majority of the water is removed. The resulting crude N_2O gas mixture is scrubbed to extract the contaminants. The gas is then compressed, dried to remove the remaining water, cooled, and liquefied. The resulting product is nearly pure (99.5% to 99.9%) and is stored as a liquefied, compressed gas at 300 psig and 4° F in insulated and refrigerated storage tanks.[1] Figure 6-1 is a flowchart of the steps involved in manufacturing, repackaging, and distributing N_2O/O_2.
  3. The manufactured product is kept refrigerated until it is directly transferred by insulated tanker trucks to hospitals with their own large storage facilities or to other gas repackagers and distributors. There are approximately 250 gas repackagers and 3200 distributors in the United States. The dental profession stores N_2O at an estimated 83,700 locations in the United States. The overall medical marketing and distribution system is very effectively and efficiently deployed in the industry.[1]
B. Users of N_2O
  1. Approximately 85% to 90% of the N_2O produced by the major manufacturing companies is used in health settings. The majority of this amount (80% to 85%) is used by hospitals to facilitate general anesthesia. The field of dentistry uses up to 10% of the N_2O in ambulatory clinics.[2]
  2. The chemical industry uses about 5% of the N_2O manufactured in the production of sodium azide, the explosive agent that inflates an automobile air bag.

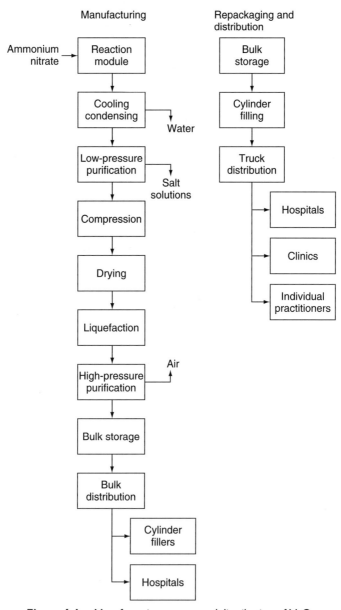

Figure 6-1   Manufacturing process and distribution of N_2O.

3. The food industry uses about 5% to 8% of the N_2O manufactured. N_2O acts as a propellant for dairy products such as whipped cream.[2]

4. N_2O is used to increase engine performance in the racing industry (i.e., cars, motorcycles, boats).[2] An N_2O system is now available for personal vehicles as well.

5. N_2O is also used in the silicon chip industry, where it oxidizes chemicals during the manufacture of computer chips. This use requires a 100% pure product.[2]

C. Manufacturers of N_2O

1. The manufacturers of N_2O are: Nellcor Puritan Bennett, Inc., Pleasanton, California; Nitrous Oxide Corporation, Radnor, Pennsylvania; Air Liquide America, Houston, Texas; and AGA, S.A. DE C.V., Mexico City.

2. Their total output is between 40 and 45 million pounds of N_2O annually.[1]

D. Product expense

1. The entire manufacturing process is very inexpensive and provides an excellent product that is affordable for both the healthcare field and industry.

2. The cost analysis of N_2O given in Chapter 7 does not include the costs of filling, storing, maintaining, or delivering the cylinders. These costs vary geographically and depend on the volume requested by the customer, the tank size, and the distance from the manufacturing site to the customer.

II. Packaging of N_2O

A. Regulatory agencies

1. The Food and Drug Administration (FDA) regulates the N_2O industry. The FDA has established Good Manufacturing Practices (GMPs) and Quality System Requirements (QSRs) with which companies who produce and package gases must comply. Compliance with these regulations results in a near 100% pure product, which exceeds U.S. Pharmacopeia specifications.

2. Additionally, the U.S. Department of Transportation (DOT) oversees the packaging and transport of the gas. N_2O is considered a hazardous material because of the pressurization. Therefore, it falls under the restrictions of the DOT Hazardous Materials Regulations. Cylinders, transportation vehicles, and drivers must meet prescribed regulations. Figure 6-2 shows a truck transporting N_2O/O_2.

B. Storing N_2O and O_2

1. Hospital settings using bulk amounts of N_2O often store the product in large containers. These containers vary in size but range from a 3¾-to a 14-ton capacity. Obviously, economic cost savings are of greatest advantage in these situations because the storage, handling, and refilling of cylinders is labor intensive.

Figure 6-2   Transportation and distribution of N_2O and O_2.

2. Most often the gas is placed into smaller storage cylinders by a local distributor for delivery.

   a. The metal cylinders are imprinted with critical information such as the origin and age of the cylinder, inspection compliance, and other important data.[2] Figure 6-3 illustrates information on the top view of typical high-pressure cylinder markings.

   b. The physical integrity of a storage cylinder determines its longevity. It is common to see cylinders 60 to 70 years old in distribution. Aluminum is an alternative cylinder material to alloy steel because of weight factors that affect regulation and cost of delivery. Small, fiberglass-wrapped cylinders offer a lightweight alternative for patients requiring ambulatory oxygen supplementation. These cylinders are the future trend in cylinder construction.

   c. Cylinders are color coded for easy identification. Color codes are uniform in the United States but may vary somewhat internationally (Table 6-1). However, the Compressed Gas Association (CGA) warns that cylinder color may not be a reliable means of gas identification. Instead, the cylinder label provides a more accurate description of the contents.[3]

   d. The size of the cylinder determines the quantity of its contents. However, depending on physical properties of the gas-liquid that is compressed into the cylinder, the amounts vary. The size of the cylinder has a direct relationship with the economy of its use. Larger cylinders are more cost effective for high-frequency use. Figure 6-4 shows examples of several different cylinder sizes. See Table 6-2 for cylinder specifications.

3. Cylinder storage is important for safety reasons as well as convenience and accessibility.

Markings prior to
January 1, 1983

Markings after
January 1, 1983

Item	Description
1	Brand identification
2	Manufacturer's test date
3	Manufacturer's registered symbol
4	Cylinder meets 10% overfill specification
5	Cylinder meets 10-year hydrostatic test exemption
6	Collar
7	Cylinder
8	Tare weight
9	D.O.T. specification and service pressure
10	Manufacturer's serial number
11	Inspector's mark
12	Registered owner (PCGCO = Nellcor Puritan Bennett)
13	Rejection elastic expansion limit in cubic centimeters

Figure 6-3   Cylinder shoulder markings detailing various information.

Table 6-1
Cylinder Color Codes for Various Countries

Country	N₂O	O₂
Australia	Blue	White
Canada	Blue	White
Germany	Gray	Blue
Sweden	Blue	White
United Kingdom	Blue	White
United States	Blue	Green
Japan	Black	White
South Africa	Blue	Black with white shoulders
Argentina	Blue	White with green cross

Table 6-2
Nitrous Oxide and Oxygen Cylinder Specifications*

Common Nitrous Oxide Cylinders

Size	Dimensions	Pressure (psig at 70° C)	Weight of N₂O	Nominal Gross Weight
D	4.25 × 17 in (10.8 × 73 cm)	745 psig	3 lb 13¼ oz (1.74 kg)	~13 lb (~2 kg)
E	4.25 × 28.75 in (10.8 × 73 cm)	745 psig	6 lb 7 oz (2.92 kg³)	~21 lb (~10 kg)
G	8.5 × 51 in (21.6 × 129.5 cm)	745 psig	56 lb (25.4 kg)	~190 lb (~86.2 kg)
H	9 × 51 in (22.9 × 129.5 cm)	745 psig	64 lb (29 kg)	~198 lb (~89.8 kg)

Common Oxygen Cylinders

Size	Pressure (psig at 70° C)	Weight of O₂	Nominal Gross Weight
D	2015 psig	15.3 ft³ (0.42 m³)	~10 lb (~4.85 kg)
E	2015 psig	24.9 ft³ (0.69 m³)	~16.5 lb (~7.48 kg)
E (aluminum)	2015 psig	24.1 ft³ (0.67 m³)	~13 lb (~6 kg)
H	2200 psig	249 ft³ (6.9 m³)	~153 lb (~70 kg)

*Courtesy Nellcor Puritan Bennett.

a. One of the most important facts to remember regarding compressed gases is that under no circumstances should grease, oil, or any other lubricating substance come in contact with the gas or gas delivery equipment. A powerful chemical reaction such as a fire or an explosion could occur. When compressed gas pressure is combined with the oxidizing property of N₂O/O₂ and an increased temperature in the reducing valve, the right conditions exist to create a potential explosion.

b. Larger cylinders associated with a central supply system are stored in an area away from the operatory. Regulations should be followed regarding ventilating and fireproofing the storage room, as well as securing and handling the cylinders.

Figure 6-4   Common gas cylinder sizes.

    c. All cylinders should be handled with care and should not be altered. They should only be handled by qualified individuals.

    d. Cylinders should be secured in a place that is not readily accessible or visible to others.

4. Requirements for appropriate cylinder storage, installation of equipment, etc., are found in Section 99-C of the National Fire Protection Association (NFPA) code. Additional information from the CGA and the National Welding Supply Association (NWSA) is available. See Appendix A for resources.

C. N_2O cylinders

   1. A full N_2O cylinder contains approximately 95% liquid and 5% vapor.

    a. Liquid N_2O in the tank is vaporized by the ambient room air temperature outside the tank as the gas is used.

    b. Because of this heat transfer process, the tank becomes cool to the touch; frost may be seen on the tank surface during prolonged and continuous use.

   2. A full cylinder of N_2O will have a pressure-gauge reading of approximately 750 psi at 70° F. If the cylinder is colder as a result of storage conditions or rapid release, the full cylinder pressure will be less. At a temperature of 50° F, the cylinder pressure will be about 575 psi.

Nitrous oxide

Oxygen

Figure 6-5   Pressure gauge readings for N_2O and O_2 cylinders.

a. Because the liquid is vaporized as the gas is used, this reading is not proportional to the actual amount of gas available in the cylinder.

b. Therefore the gauge will show a pressure decrease when the tank contains approximately 20% N$_2$O. The drop in the dial on the N$_2$O tank is not proportional to the contents of the tank as with O$_2$. Figure 6-5 illustrates pressure gauge readings for full and empty N$_2$O and O$_2$ cylinders.

D. O$_2$ cylinders

1. O$_2$ is found as a gas in a cylinder. When the O$_2$ cylinder is full, the amount of pressure is approximately 2000 psi.

2. The pressure gauge for O$_2$ will accurately indicate the amount of gas present in the cylinder at all times until the cylinder is exhausted.

a. The dial will accurately reflect the quantity of gas available in the cylinder for use. For example, if the dial reads 1000 psi, the cylinder is considered half full.

b. It is important to monitor the amount of O$_2$ left in the cylinder while it is in use. Because the N$_2$O/O$_2$ sedation machine is driven by O$_2$ flow, if the O$_2$ tank becomes empty during a procedure, there will be no flow of N$_2$O and the sedation experience will be interrupted. It is important to have additional O$_2$ cylinders available to prevent this occurrence.

III. Manufacturers of N$_2$O/O$_2$ Sedation Equipment

A. There are three major companies in the United States that manufacture and distribute N$_2$O/O$_2$ delivery systems. They are, in alphabetical order: Accutron, Inc., Phoenix, Arizona; Matrx Medical Inc., Orchard Park, New York; and Porter Instrument Co., Inc., Hatfield, Pennsylvania. (See Appendix A for references.)

B. *Authors' note:* We can personally attest to the genuine concern of each of these companies to manufacture the best and safest products for the mutual benefit of both patient and professional.

IV. Delivery of N$_2$O/O$_2$

A. History and evolution of N$_2$O/O$_2$ delivery equipment

1. N$_2$O/O$_2$ sedation equipment has evolved dramatically since the initial delivery through a bladder bag for Horace Wells.

2. Sir Fredrick Hewitt in 1887 was the first to incorporate oxygen into a machine that delivered both gases.[4]

3. Early machines were designed as intermittent (demand) flow.[4]

4. A pivotal point in the progression of this technology was the addition of the fail-safe O$_2$ mechanism in the mid-1970s. This device prevented the delivery of 100% N$_2$O and ensured that no less than 21% O$_2$ (O$_2$ concentration in ambient air) would ever be delivered to the patient.[3] Today this tolerance is 30%.

5. Mr. Gary Porter, President of Porter Instrument Co., Inc., played an integral role in the evolution of the early analgesia-sedation units. The Porter Instrument Co. is the only company to manufacture the flowmeter glass tubes found in sedation units and hospital anesthesia machines around the world.

6. Today we enjoy the amenities of audible alarms, digital readouts, tactile-sensitive features, and high-quality performance.

B. Central gas supply system

1. A central gas supply system is used when a large quantity of gas is - supplying several units. Practitioners may prefer this system because of the frequency of N_2O/O_2 use, cost savings, convenience, space saving, etc.

2. A central-system manifold (Figure 6-6) is a device that connects several large cylinders of gas together and allows for the transfer of gas supply from one tank to another when the tank is depleted.

a. A manifold is used to connect a central gas supply to individual operatories and to ensure a constant availability of gas.

Figure 6-6   Central manifold system. (Courtesy Matrx Medical, Inc.)

b. A manifold system can be manually operated or virtually self-automated.

c. Manifold systems are designed to supply gas to as many as 10 units in a given facility. Beyond 10 units, the facility is considered a hospital-care unit and is regulated accordingly.

d. The manifold system is most conveniently and effectively used when it is incorporated as part of the architectural design of the operatory (Figure 6-7).

e. The newest manifolds have several safety features built into the system.

   i. Pressure-relief valves exhaust any gas higher than 75 psi.

   ii. Alarm systems, both visual and audible, alert a designated person if the pressure of the gas falls below 45 psi or becomes higher than 60 psi. A wall alarm placed in the operatory alerts the practitioner, whereas a desk alarm alerts an individual at a central location (Figure 6-8).

3. All gas from the manifold travels through precleaned, degreased copper tubing, and all connections are silver-soldered at 1000° F. The piping system must be pressure tested with N_2 (air) for 24 hours at no less than 150 psi before patient use. Half-inch copper tubing for delivery of O_2 and ⅜-inch tubing for N_2O have become norms. The difference in tubing size prohibits the inadvertent crossing of lines. However, at least one fatality has occurred because of installation errors and subsequent delivery of 100% N_2O instead of O_2. Piping, Industry, Progress, and Education (PIPE) is an organization dedicated to educating users of N_2O/O_2 seda-

Typical System Layout

Operatory
One outlet station per operatory.

Zone valve
Required when tank room is in a remote location.

Reception area

Tank room
• Storage of tanks
• Manifold
• Regulators
• Tank restrainers
• Instructions
• Hose connections
• Ventilated
• Fire-proof door

Reception office
Alarm indicators in desk or wall models

Figure 6-7   Examples of office configuration using a central manifold system.

Figure 6-8 Two types of alarm systems. **A,** Wall mounted (Courtesy Matrx Medical, Inc.) and **B,** desk mounted.

CGA Connection No. 326   **CGA Connection No. 540**

Figure 6-9   Large cylinder threaded valve connections.

tion about the proper installation of the system. See Appendix A for references.

4. For the gas to be dispensed safely there must be a means for reducing the amount of gas pressure from the cylinder. A pressure-reducing valve or regulator is necessary to ensure safe delivery of gas to the patient and through the equipment.

a. The high pressures of 750 psi in the N_2O tank and 2000 psi in the O_2 tank are reduced to lower pressures of approximately 50 psi.

b. Regulators are commonly found on or near the cylinders of central supply delivery systems.

c. Pressure gauges accompany regulators and display gas pressures within the tank. Pressure gauges indicating the amount of pressure in the lines may also be present on a central manifold system.

5. Large G and H cylinders are used in central supply systems. There is a safety feature within the threaded valves that open the cylinders. Threaded stems are designed to fit into specific cylinders only, thus preventing the cylinders being filled with the wrong gas (Figure 6-9).

C. Portable gas delivery system

1. A portable gas delivery system is often used when N_2O/O_2 sedation is not used frequently. The unit houses smaller tanks and may be moved easily from place to place.

2. The yoke stand of the portable machine is the backbone and supporting structure upon which the equipment rests. Stands vary slightly in style; all are easily transportable on wheels. Some stands hold two tanks whereas others hold four tanks (Figure 6-10). One company markets a portable system that encloses the yoke and tanks for easy maneuverability (Figure 6-11).

3. The yoke is the metal framework adjoining the stand to which the cylinders are attached. There is an attachment configuration for the cylinder to

A

B

Figure 6-10   Two- and four-cylinder portable yoke stands. (Courtesy Accutron, Inc.)

Figure 6-11   Encased portable yoke and tanks. (Courtesy Accutron, Inc.)

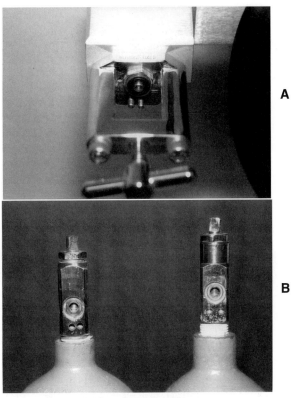

Figure 6-12   Pin index safety system.

match to be correctly attached to the unit. Metal pins, specifically arranged, protrude from the yoke onto which the cylinder is fitted (Figure 6-12). This precise mechanism is designed to prevent the incorrect cylinder attachment to the yoke and is known as the *pin index safety system* (Figure 6-13).

4. Regulators are found on portable systems similar to central delivery systems (Figure 6-14). After the gas pressure has been reduced, gas is delivered through low-pressure hosing connected to the back of the flowmeter, the boxlike portion of the unit, which contains switches, knobs, etc. (Figure 6-15). These hoses are color coded respectively for the gases and purposely vary in size and threaded end connections to prevent improper gas flow to the machine.

5. At this point, the equipment is the same whether delivering gas from a central supply or a portable unit.

D. Flowmeter

1. The flowmeter is the highly calibrated device that sits on top of the yoke assembly, is mounted to the wall, or is located within the cabinetry (Figure 6-16). Gas flows from the cylinder through the flowmeter. The flowmeter indicates the amount of gas being delivered to the patient.

Post type valve with pin-indexed outlet

CGA Connection No. 870
Valve yoke
connection oxygen

CGA Connection No. 910
Medical cylinder valve
connection nitrous oxide

Figure 6-13 Small tank pin index system.

2. Gas flows into separate sections of the flowmeter and ultimately shows its flow in the gas tubes on the front of the unit. Small balls within the tubes rise and fall according to the amount of gas flowing into the flowmeter. The number corresponding to the middle of the ball indicates the liters of flow per minute of a gas being delivered to the patient. Digital lighted electronic displays are also available. In this case, flashing lights indicate the flow of gas (Figure 6-17).

3. One of the most important safety features of the sedation unit is the flowmeter's fail-safe mechanism. A valve opens to allow N_2O flow only when there is flow of O_2 to the system. Any time the O_2 flow is less than 30%, N_2O stops flowing. This feature prevents the potential delivery of

Figure 6-14   Regulators alter high pressure from cylinders to low pressure for patient delivery.

Figure 6-15   Pressure hosing from regulators into flowmeter.

100% N$_2$O and is standard on every sedation unit made today. *Without it, an operator is practicing below the standard of care.* See Figure 6-18 for specific features of the flowmeter.

E. Reservoir bag

  1. The reservoir bag (Figure 6-19) serves three purposes. Its primary purpose is to provide a source of additional gas should the patient inspire more gas than is being supplied through the hoses. Typically, a reservoir bag holds approximately 3 L of gas. Other sizes are available (e.g., a smaller bag for pediatric patients).

Figure 6-16   A, Flowmeter on top of yoke assembly. **B,** Flowmeter mounted to wall. **C,** Flowmeter located within cabinetry. (Courtesy Porter Instrument Co., Inc.)

Figure 6-17   Digital LED flowmeter. (Courtesy Matrx Medical, Inc.)

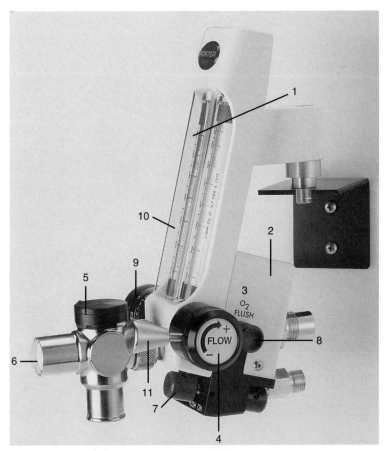

Figure 6-18   Flowmeter features. *1*, Flowmeter tubes; *2*, fail-safe; *3*, gas control block; *4*, gas flow adjustment knobs; *5*, emergency air valve; *6*, check valve (nonrebreathing valve); *7*, positive ON-OFF switch; *8*, oxygen flush button; *9*, needle valves; *10*, flowmeter; *11*, total flow adjustment knob. (Courtesy Porter Instrument Co., Inc.)

Figure 6-19   Reservoir bag.

Figure 6-20   Conduction tubing connected to scavenging nasal hood.
(Courtesy Accutron, Inc.)

2. Additionally, the reservoir bag provides a mechanism for monitoring the patient's respiration. Watching the expansion and contraction of the bag during sedation assures the operator of the patient's quiet inhalation and exhalation.

3. The reservoir bag also functions in an emergency as a method of providing positive-pressure O_2 to the patient. The bag is gently squeezed to empty its contents into the pulmonary tree; the action is similar to a manual-resuscitator bag. Assisting ventilation in this manner overcomes resistance when accompanied by a full face mask with a tight seal rather than a nasal hood.

Figure 6-21   Scavenging nasal hoods in a variety of sizes. (Courtesy Matrx Medical, Inc.)

F. Conduction tubing
  1. Gas is delivered through tubing or hose stemming from the unit and attaching to the breathing apparatus, as shown in Figure 6-20.
  2. Care should be taken to prevent kinking of the hose, thereby preventing gas flow. If this should happen the patient will most likely alert the operator of breathing difficulty. The reservoir bag will also overfill and balloon because of the constriction of the hose.
  3. The concept of anatomic dead space is relative to the length of the conduction tubing. This space will contain gas that neither gets into the pulmonary tree to be utilized nor is expelled from the system to be replaced by fresh gas, hence "dead space." The distance from the gas source to the patient's lungs can increase the anatomic dead space and be lengthened by the conduction tubing. It is important not to add hose to facilitate delivery to another area or the other side of the room because of this factor.
  4. Units may consist of a combination of corrugated and noncorrugated tubing. Tubing diameters vary, with most tubing narrowing near the attachment of the breathing apparatus.
G. Breathing apparatus (nasal hood or face mask)
  1. Gas may be delivered to the patient through a nasal hood or a full face mask. Depending on the discipline, one method may be favored over the other. For example, in dentistry, because of the necessity of access to the mouth, a full face mask is not practical.
  2. The nasal hood is most commonly used with today's sedation equipment. One of the reasons for this is that dentistry represents a large sample of the product consumers.
    a. The nasal hood is designed to fit snugly over the patient's nose so that gas does not leak out the sides. There are several sizes available (Figure 6-21).

Figure 6-22   Scavenging nasal hoods in a variety of scents. (Courtesy Accutron, Inc.)

Figure 6-23   Some scavenging nasal hoods are sterilizable and can be reused. (Courtesy Porter Instrument Co., Inc.)

b. Hoods are offered in a variety of scents such as vanilla, peach, strawberry, mint, and bubble gum (Figure 6-22). Unscented nasal hoods are also available.

c. The most current models of nasal hoods are designed for single patient use. Many regard these as disposable because they are not sterilizable. Other reusable versions of the hoods are also available but must be sterilized between patients (Figure 6-23).

d. Practitioners may choose to dispose of the nasal hood and recover the cost in the sedation fee or sell the nasal hood to patients and suggest they bring it to the next appointment.

e. All nasal hoods should have scavenging capabilities. Scavenging nasal hoods are designed to provide fresh gas to the hood for the patient through two hoses while one or two additional hoses evacuate gas being exhaled by the patient (see Figure 6-20). These hoses are connected to a vacuum system that exhausts the gases out of the building.

f. *It is considered practicing below the standard of care for any healthcare professional not to use a scavenging nasal hood.*

3. A full face mask may be used in place of the nasal hood when accessibility to the mouth is not an issue. A piece of elastic usually accompanies the mask and is placed over the patient's head to secure the mask. Because the mask is intended to cover both the mouth and nose, it is much larger than the nasal hood. Patients may remark that it is claustrophobic by design and may be more anxious about its placement. It is generally used for anesthetic procedures (i.e., general anesthesia) or emergency oxygen delivery.

V. Variations of Equipment

A. Design
1. Currently, there are a variety of available designs of sedation equipment from which to choose. Manufacturers determine their own style, color, size, etc., of equipment. However, the design features are similar. Each has common performance features and similar safety features; any variations are in location of the features on the equipment and whether they are manual or automatic.

2. A sedation unit may have separate controls (Figure 6-24), one regulating the flow of N₂O and another controlling O₂ flow. In this case, both knobs will be used as the gases are delivered.

3. Another type of unit (Figure 6-25) may be able to mix the gases together and control the total flow being delivered to a patient. This unit is designed to maintain a constant total flow to the patient; gas is increased or decreased using one dial. The percentage of N₂O administered can be adjusted with the dial.

4. Matrx Medical has designed a sedation unit that includes an LED panel (Figure 6-26) and an audible alarm system. The mixing unit is controlled with arrow keys for increasing or decreasing gas, and it can maintain a

Figure 6-24   Sedation unit with separate gas flow controls. (Courtesy Accutron, Inc.)

Figure 6-25   Sedation unit capable of mixing gases and maintaining constant tidal volume. (Courtesy Accutron, Inc.)

constant liters flow. This machine has many advantages such as automaticity and precision of gas flow.

5. The Ultra flowmeter, designed by Accutron, Inc., has the capability of blocking the flow of N_2O with a lock. This feature maintains the value of the machine as an O_2-delivering mechanism in emergency situations while simultaneously securing the N_2O (see Figure 6-25).

Figure 6-26   Digital LED panel controlled with arrow keys. (Courtesy Matrx Medical, Inc.)

6. An international manufacturer in Japan produces a machine that calculates the amount of N_2O and O_2 used for a procedure. The cost of N_2O is quite high ($20 per pound) in Japan. Consumers are charged for the exact amount (per gram) of N_2O used. The machine displays the amount and subsequent charge to the patient on a receiptlike slip of paper for direct reimbursement to the healthcare facility (see Chapter 7).

B. Customization
   1. Depending on specific consumer needs, manufacturers can customize equipment accordingly.
   2. Restrictions may apply regarding the maximum allowable N_2O concentrations able to be administered by some groups, countries, or organizations. Certain military groups regulate concentrations and thus purchase units that have been customized to limit the amount of N_2O able to be delivered.
   3. Equipment available for international use varies widely. Depending on the country using the sedation equipment, markings may be customized to accommodate various languages; colored hoses, tubing, etc., may vary depending on the color codes specific to a country.

C. Cost
   1. The cost of the necessary sedation equipment should not be prohibitive to providing this service. Expenses will be recovered quickly with patient use and reimbursement of fees.
   2. As mentioned earlier, it is necessary to choose the delivery mode according to the frequency of use. A central system is much more cost effective; it should be included in building plans if frequent use is expected. The portable system offers the flexibility of moving from place to place without the initial expense.
   3. Although initial costs for the central system are much greater than for the portable system, the use of N_2O provides economic benefit. The greater

initial cost of the central system can be recovered in a short time. See Chapter 7 for information regarding economic benefits.

D. Maintenance

1. Manufacturers recommend servicing sedation units periodically. Each company may have specific time frames for maintenance of its units. It is prudent to follow these recommendations to ensure safe delivery to the patient.

2. Servicing a unit includes procedures such as recalibration, pressure testing, internal component checking and replacement, and other factory testing procedures.

3. If at any time the integrity of the equipment is questionable or the unit is not functioning properly, it is important to discontinue its use and alert those who service the equipment. Unqualified personnel must not be allowed to tamper with or attempt to repair any sedation equipment. Servicing and inspecting must be left to those that are properly trained.

VI. Equipment Safety Features

A. Several safety features are inherent components of N_2O/O_2 delivery equipment for ambulatory settings. These features provide both patient and professional assurance of the safe delivery of N_2O/O_2 sedation.

1. The most important safety feature of the unit is the O_2 fail-safe mechanism. It ensures that N_2O will not be delivered unless there is O_2 flowing to the machine. Because of this device, the possibility of administering 100% N_2O to a patient has been eliminated. The mechanism's function is based on pressure. O_2 flows into the unit at a pressure that opens a valve to allow the flow of N_2O. If the O_2 pressure drops because of depletion of the supply, the valve closes, thereby preventing the flow of N_2O. This safety feature is standard on every sedation unit manufactured today. Units made before 1976, when this feature was added, should not be used. Using outdated equipment places operators in legal jeopardy because they are practicing below the established standard of care.

2. Currently, the units manufactured in the United States are designed to deliver a minimum of 30% O_2 at all times. It is critical to maintain an O_2 level of at least that in ambient air (21%). The minimum of 30% established by the manufacturers allows for a margin of error in calibration. Similarly, the equipment is designed to deliver no more than 70% N_2O at any time. For analgesia and sedation purposes, it is not necessary to administer N_2O concentrations higher than 70%.

3. An index safety system is designed to prevent the inadvertent attachment of the N_2O cylinder to an O_2 portal.

   a. A pin system is used for portable machines in which small cylinders attach to the yoke. Each cylinder of compressed gas has two small holes drilled into the valve stem that correspond to a specific configuration identifying the contents of the cylinder. Two small pins on each portal of the yoke configured exactly with the holes on the cylinder form the attachment mechanism between the cylinder and unit (see Figure 6-12).

b. On equipment that uses larger tanks, the index system includes thread size and configuration of the valve connection on the tank to the regulator. Again, each gas has a specific configuration to avoid incorrect attachments (see Figure 6-9).

4. With the diameter index safety system, the hoses through which the gas travels from the cylinder to the unit are unable to be attached to the wrong stem. The attachment couplings are different in diameter, as are the hoses and stems (Figure 6-27).

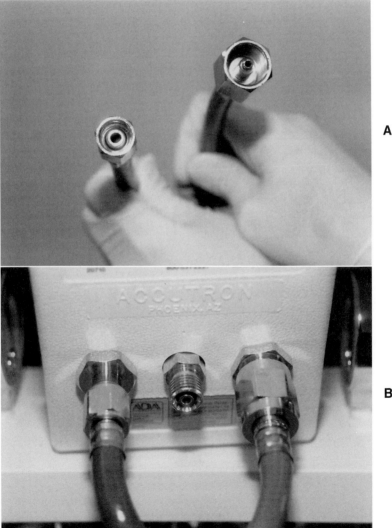

Figure 6-27   **A,** Note the difference in diameter of the attachment couplings in the diameter safety system. **B,** Diameter index safety system.

Figure 6-28   Positive-pressure oxygen connection.

Figure 6-29   Quick-connect bag and mask for emergency situations. (Courtesy Porter Instrument Co., Inc.)

5. Near the unit's reservoir bag is an emergency air inlet. This provides an additional source of air for the patient in the circumstance that the reservoir bag is inadequate or the gas flow decreases for some reason (see Figure 6-18).
6. A nonrebreathing valve located near the reservoir bag prohibits exhaled gas from the tubing from entering the reservoir bag (see Figure 6-18).
7. The reservoir bag may serve to assist with patient respirations should an emergency situation arise.
8. There is an auxiliary positive-pressure oxygen hookup on the unit (Figure 6-28) capable of accommodating a quick-connect bag and mask (Figure 6-29). The sedation unit is indispensable for emergency resuscitation situations.
9. There are several alarm options, depending on the type of system or unit being used. Alarms can be audible and/or visual to indicate a depleting oxygen supply. Audible alarms are mandatory in Europe and are recommended in the United States.

REFERENCES

1. Fettes WC: Personal communication, August 1996.
2. *Compressed Gas Association code-201, nitrous oxide sales and security recommended guidelines*, Arlington, Va, 1995, Compressed Gas Association.
3. *Compressed Gas Association code-9, standard color marking of compressed gas containers intended for medical use*, Arlington, Va, 1993, Compressed Gas Association.
4. Malamed SF: *Sedation: a guide to patient management*, ed 4, St Louis, 2003, Mosby.

7

Economic Benefits Associated with N_2O/O_2 Administration

When the subject of economics enters the realm of patient care, many practitioners begin to feel uneasy. Although financial expectations may not be the centerpiece of a decision to pursue a health career, they often are a significant factor. Being financially successful is not unethical by itself, although there are those in the medical profession who have abused the system for financial gain. However, there is nothing wrong with caring about people and enjoying the benefits of success. Health professionals should feel good about the services they provide and be profitable enough to continue to practice them.

I. Economic Reflection

A. The "Golden Age of Medicine and Dentistry," a period of post-World War II prosperity that lasted into the early 1960s, was a time of high demand for services and a shortage of clinicians. This situation assured professionals that their practices would be profitable. Because patients were waiting at the door, schedules became tight and profits became palpable. Unfortunately, time and compassion for the patient were not as important for many as they should have been.
B. As the supply of practitioners began to increase in the early 1970s, the demand for healthcare professionals decreased, as did the patient-to-practitioner ratio.
C. Renewed interest in the relationship between clinician and patient has demanded greater sensitivity to patient problems, payment plans, and scheduling demands, and an overall awareness of patient needs.

II. Realistic Economics

A. Today's patients have a greater choice in the overall environment of treatment. If they are not treated considerately in one office, they can more easily than ever find an office that makes a greater effort toward meeting their individual needs. This is the basic economic principle of supply and demand in action. Caring, compassionate, competent practitioners are doing very well and have not had economic setbacks because of "too much competition." Indeed, choice has led to patient sophistication in consumerism.

B. Regardless of the socioeconomic strata or educational profiles of patients, they as human beings can easily, quickly, and accurately recognize the sincerity of a clinician. Based on experiences, patients use their intuition to determine whether they will continue with a certain doctor and whether they will refer others to that doctor. Patients do not necessarily have the ability to evaluate a clinician's technical or decision-making skills; therefore their evaluations are based on the clinicians' personal interactions with them.

C. With the advent of managed care, health maintenance organizations (HMOs), preferred provider organization (PPO) programs, and changing insurance issues, practitioners' knowledge and understanding of economics becomes critical to survival. Clearly, ambulatory services have and will continue to increase because of the regulations placed on time, payments, extent of treatment, etc. Many practitioners feel that these issues have become so intrusive that patient care has suffered.

D. Overall change in medicine. There is no doubt that medicine is changing. Practitioners are being challenged to find new avenues for providing patient care with renewed compassion. They may have to advocate services in a different manner. Practitioners may have to rethink their commitment to the profession and to the patient. They may have to become innovative in treatment planning.

E. Patient-driven practices. Patients are always grateful for honest and sincere efforts. In time they will demand the return of lost services and individual decision-making. They will stand behind those professionals they trust. Practices are truly patient driven.

III. Dollars and "Sense"

A. Do you consider your patients' comfort levels valuable? Are you less stressed because you have relaxed, cooperative patients? If so, how much money is that worth? Although these and other rhetorical questions may be intangible, a more concrete question is "How much money can you truly save or earn using N_2O/O_2 sedation in your practice?" Box 7-1 shows the income potential of using N_2O/O_2 sedation.

B. The actual cost savings or moneymaking potential of using N_2O/O_2 sedation varies with certain factors. Patient numbers will increase, and time efficiency will be enhanced. These factors alone will increase bottom-line figures proportionally.

   1. An initial decision must be made as to what type of N_2O/O_2 system will be the most beneficial and cost effective. Table 7-1 compares the central gas supply system with the portable gas supply system.

      a. Obviously, if N_2O/O_2 sedation will be common practice in a particular setting, a central supply system should be considered.

         i. This system allows for multiple flowmeters to be placed in several rooms. Piping and connecting are done within the structure; therefore moving machines and hoses from room to room is not necessary.

BOX 7-1
Income Potential Using N$_2$O/O$_2$ Sedation

N_2O at $50 per visit
Weekly:
Twice per week	=	$100
Once per day	=	$250
Twice per day	=	$500

Monthly:
Twice per week monthly	=	$400
Once per day monthly	=	$1000
Twice per day monthly	=	$2000

Yearly:
Once per day	=	$12,000

NOTE: Average fee for N$_2$O (short procedure) is $50.00. Figures based on E-cylinders.

ii. This type of system allows for larger quantities of gas to be stored in a remote location. Larger cylinders, capable of storing more gas, are much less expensive per unit of gas than smaller ones.
b. Individual, portable units are also available. Practitioners may choose this option as personal preference, especially when only occasionally using N$_2$O/O$_2$ and when confines of the physical structure do not allow for a central system.
    i. The entire portable system is on a rolling stand and may be moved from room to room.
    ii. Gas cylinders for this type of system are smaller, store less gas, and are more expensive per unit of gas than gas cylinders for central systems.

Table 7-1
Central Gas Supply System versus Portable Gas Supply System

	Portable System		Central System
Cylinders used	Small E tanks		Large G (N$_2$O) or H (O$_2$) tanks
Cylinder volume	9 E tanks (N$_2$O)	in	1 G tank (N$_2$O)
	10 E tanks (O$_2$)	in	1 H tank (O$_2$)
Approximate cost to have filled	$12 (N$_2$O)		$48.00 (N$_2$O)
	$6 (O$_2$)		$11.00 (O$_2$)

If the clinic uses 10 G (N$_2$O) cylinders and 20 H (O$_2$) cylinders in 1 year, the savings from using large cylinders would be:

	N$_2$O		O$_2$
E tanks:	(9 × $12 × 10)	+	(10 × $6 × 20) = $2280
G and H tanks:	($48 × 10)	+	($11 × 20) = $700
			Savings = $1580 per year

NOTE: Comparison made for U.S. Coast Guard clinic with 10 operatories.

c. In either situation the initial cost of the N$_2$O/O$_2$ equipment should not be a prohibiting factor for its use. This investment will be quickly recovered.

2. The cost of N$_2$O and O$_2$ gases varies considerably in terms of size and quantity of cylinders ordered and distance from a distribution center. Depending on location, costs increase proportionally to the levels of individuals involved with distributorship. Gas costs will most likely be higher the further the distance from a distributor (Figure 7-1).

3. Patient charges for N$_2$O/O$_2$ sedation vary dramatically. They can range from $15 per visit to $80 per visit.

   a. Some professionals do not charge the patient for N$_2$O/O$_2$ sedation but rather include it in the overall fee for service to the patient.

   b. Insurance companies vary as to their payment policies for this service. It is wise to investigate what is considered to be the usual and customary fee according to your most common insurance carriers and local practitioners.

   c. In Japan, an N$_2$O/O$_2$ machine has the ability to determine the amount of gas delivered to the patient in terms of "flow time." The charge to the patient is calculated according to the cost of the gas mul-

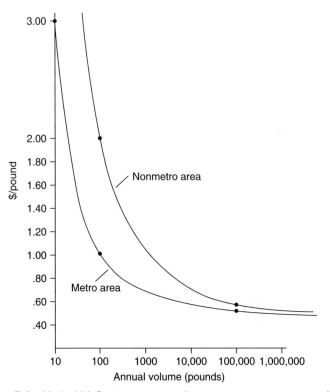

Figure 7-1   Medical N$_2$O pricing, metropolitan areas versus nonmetropolitan areas.

Figure 7-2 N_2O/O_2 machine capable of calculating patient charges according to the amount of gas used. (Courtesy Dr. Yuzuru Kaneko, Dept. of Dental Anesthesiology, Tokyo Dental College, Tokyo, Japan.)

tiplied by the amount of gas used. The machine is capable of printing out a charge slip for the patient at each visit (Figure 7-2).

C. Although dollar figures vary between individual situations, N_2O/O_2 sedation is profitable. Figures relating to profit in goodwill from acknowledging and diminishing patients' anxiety should not be discounted. Profit is also made by patient referrals. In economic jargon, this is a win-win situation. It just makes sense.

PART II
ANATOMY, PHYSIOLOGY, AND ADMINISTRATION

8

Anatomy and Physiology of Respiration and Airway Management

Any method of inhalation sedation involves those anatomic structures associated with the inhalation and exhalation of air and the exchange of gases. To integrate the pharmacologic properties of N_2O into a clinical setting, the basic principles of the anatomy and physiology of respiration should be reviewed.

I. Respiratory System Design and Function

A. Design. The respiratory system is primarily designed to perform the function of exchanging gases—functionally carbon dioxide (CO_2) and O_2—across pulmonary capillary membranes. The design of the system allows this function to be performed continuously and with minimal effort by the body.[1]
B. Function. Respiration is driven automatically by the brainstem (medulla oblongata) and voluntarily by the cerebral cortex.[2]

II. Anatomy of the Upper Airway

A. Nose
   1. The respiratory functions of the nose are to warm incoming air to body temperature, humidify the air, and filter macroparticles via nose hair and microparticles via cilia.
   2. Because the nose is also a primary entrance of gases used during inhalation sedation, it is critical to the effectiveness of the procedure that a patient is able to breathe well. Anatomic conditions affecting air passage through the nose (e.g., a deviated septum, enlarged tonsils and adenoids) may interfere with N_2O/O_2 delivery.
B. Pharynx
   1. The pharynx is a cylindric, muscular tube about 12 to 14 cm long.
   2. It is divided into three sections (Figure 8-1): the nasopharynx, oropharynx, and laryngopharynx.
      a. The nasopharynx is located behind the nasal cavity. The adenoids, tonsils, and openings to the eustachian tubes are found here. The soft palate separates the nasopharynx from the oropharynx.
      b. The oropharynx opens into the mouth and serves as the link between the nasopharynx and the laryngopharynx. It serves as an entrance to

Figure 8-1   Nasopharynx, oropharynx, and laryngopharynx. (From Thibodeau GA, Patton KT: *The human body in health and disease*, ed 3, St Louis, 2002, Mosby.)

the larynx and esophagus. Its boundaries are the soft palate and the epiglottis at the level of the hyoid bone. The epiglottis is connected by the medial glossoepiglottic fold and bilateral glossoepiglottic fold. These folds create a depression called the *valleculae*. Lateral to this central area on either side is a piriform recess. These recesses are the common location for collecting foreign objects, thereby protecting the lower airway.

c. The laryngopharynx begins at the epiglottis. The epiglottis is the cartilaginous, leaf-shaped structure that projects upward behind the tongue. This flaplike structure (Figure 8-2) directs material backward to the esophagus and prevents objects from entering the trachea during swallowing. The laryngopharynx extends from the epiglottis to the cricoid cartilage. The larynx lies inside the laryngopharynx. The framework of the laryngopharynx is made up of the thyroid cartilage, which is shaped like a shield, and the cricoid cartilage, which is ring shaped. Several muscle groups and ligaments cover these large structures. Both cartilages offer significant protection to the underlying larynx.

III. Anatomy of the Lower Airway

A. Larynx
   1. The air passageway continues with the larynx. Pearl-colored vocal cords are housed here, which, when vibrated with air, produce vocal sound. The glottal opening at the vocal cords is the narrowest part of the adult airway; the cricoid ring is the narrowest part of the pediatric (younger than 7 to 10 years of age) airway.
   2. Strong muscles (false vocal cords) that adduct to prevent entry of foreign objects protect the sensitive mucosa of the larynx. If the larynx is irritated, the defensive cough reflex is initiated. Coughing occurs when high pressure is produced in the lower respiratory tract by the closing of the epiglottis and vocal cords and the contracting of expiratory and abdominal muscles. A sudden opening of the false vocal cords allows the air to explode out of the respiratory tract, carrying the foreign matter with it.[2] It is important to note that the use of N_2O for inhalation sedation allows this vital defensive reflex to remain intact.
B. Trachea
   1. The trachea, a muscular tube contiguous with the larynx, begins at the sixth cervical vertebra and is surrounded by horseshoe-shaped cartilaginous rings. It is approximately 11 cm long with a lumen size of approximately 20 mm. Figure 8-3 shows the trachea and bronchi.

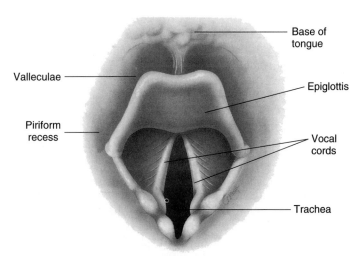

Base of tongue

Valleculae

Epiglottis

Piriform recess

Vocal cords

Trachea

Figure 8-2   Larynx and epiglottis. (From Thibodeau GA, Patton KT: *The human body in health and disease*, ed 3, St Louis, 2002, Mosby.)

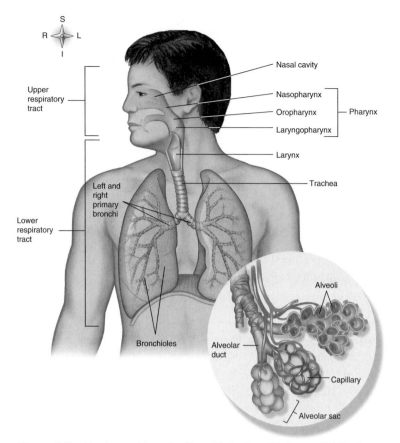

Figure 8-3 Trachea and bronchi. (From Thibodeau GA, Patton KT: *The human body in health and disease*, ed 3, St Louis, 2002, Mosby.)

2. The trachea bifurcates asymmetrically into the right and left bronchi. A highly sensitive, neurologically rich area, the carina (Figure 8-4), marks this bifurcation. The carina is considered a back-up defense mechanism for the cough reflex. If an object passes through the first defense site (larynx), the carina causes the defensive cough to continue. Submucosal swelling and partial obstruction in this area can result from a strong stimulus and lead to severe airway resistance.

C. Bronchi

1. The right bronchus is approximately 2.5 cm long and deviates slightly from the trachea at approximately 25 degrees. Because of the minimal divergence from the trachea, aspirated foreign objects are more commonly directed to the right lung. Comparatively, the left bronchus is twice as long and smaller in diameter than its right counterpart. It deviates closer to 45 degrees from the trachea (see Figure 8-4).

2. The main stem bronchi diverge into smaller branches responsible for the upper, middle, and lower lobes of the lung. The right bronchus divides into three branches, which link to three upper lobes, two middle lobes,

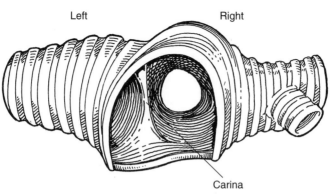

Figure 8-4   Carina located at the bifurcation of the bronchi.

and five lower lobes. The left bronchus bifurcates into two branches that give rise to five upper lobes and four lower lobes. Each lobe contains conducting and respiratory bronchioli with dependent alveolar ducts, sacs, and alveoli.

D. Bronchioles
   1. Bronchioles are a continued division of the bronchi but are identified by the lack of cartilage.
   2. The first 16 of the 23 generations of bronchiole divisions are considered conducting airways in normal anatomy.[2] These airways are incapable of exchanging gases. At generation 17 the respiratory bronchioli begin the respiratory zone. These are smaller than the parent bronchioli but contain significantly more surface area.[2]

IV. Anatomy of the Respiratory Zone

A. Bronchioli, alveolar ducts, alveolar sacs, and alveoli
   1. Alveolar ducts mark the transition between bronchioli, alveolar sacs, and alveoli, as shown in Figure 8-3.
   2. Alveolar sacs "pouch" to form the thin-walled alveoli.
   3. It is in the 300 million alveoli of an adult that the exchange between air and blood takes place.[2]

V. Physiology of the Respiratory Mechanism

A. The medullary center in the brainstem controls the automatic respiratory process of breathing. Active inspiration is accomplished principally by the diaphragm and external intercostal muscles and assisted by the scalenes and sternocleidomastoids. As the diaphragm moves downward, the chest wall expands, creating negative pressure in the pleural space, thereby allowing a vacuum effect to pull air into the system. This motion, producing a drop in air pressure in the lungs, provides the principal mechanics for inspiration.

B. Air continues to flow until pressures from inside the lung are equivalent to atmospheric pressure. Expiration occurs passively as the chest wall and lungs recoil. This recoil causes another pressure change in which the compressed air is quietly pushed out of the lungs. Expiration becomes active only when changes in respiratory demands such as exercise, abnormalities, or disease occur. This automatic, regular ebb-and-flow movement of air is called *tidal flow* because of its similarities to that of the ocean tide.[2]

C. Because of the pressure gradient that exists between the lung walls and the thoracic cavity, the lungs are distended and fill the cavity while atmospheric pressure pushes the chest wall inward. The fluid between the structures prevents the two from separating. If air enters the pleural cavity, as in a trauma, a pneumothorax results. The fluid holding the lungs against the wall cannot hold the two together.

D. The amount of gas inspired into the lungs (tidal volume) depends largely on the physical characteristics of the individual (Figure 8-5). Generally, larger chest cavities hold more volume than smaller chest cavities. Males' lung volumes are approximately 25% greater than those of females in general.[3]

   1. In a normal-size adult of average physical ability and without lung disease, the tidal volume approaches 500 ml. Minute ventilation (volume) is the amount of gas brought into the lungs each minute. It is calculated by multiplying the tidal volume by the rate of respiration (e.g., 500 ml × 12 to 15 respirations per minute = approximately 6 to 7 L per minute).[1-3]

   2. Minute ventilation is significant in terms of N_2O administration because it deals with how much gas mixture (N_2O/O_2) should be given to a patient. Inadequate amounts are likely to produce a suffocating feeling and make the act of breathing laborious. Conversely, too much gas forced into the nasal hood of the delivery system will cause some to be wasted. Because it is not being consumed by the patient, it will escape. This excess airflow not only blows into the patient's eyes, causing dryness, but also exposes personnel to unnecessary amounts of trace gas.

   3. Alveolar ventilation is the amount of air per minute entering the alveolar units capable of gas-blood exchange. This volume is less than the minute volume because not all of the inspired air reaches the alveoli during inspiration. A portion of the inhaled air occupies the conducting airways and does not enter the lungs and therefore is not taken up into the exhaust system. Hence this air is not able to participate in the gas-blood exchange. This is known as *anatomic dead space*. Therefore alveolar ventilation is calculated by subtracting the dead space volume (approximately 150 ml) from the tidal volume and then multiplying by the respiration rate.[3]

E. The critical gas exchange from alveolus to capillary and vice versa occurs through simple diffusion across partial-pressure gradients.

   1. Atmospheric air is composed of 79% N_2, 21% O_2, and 0.04% CO_2. Other gases are negligible (Box 8-1). Combined, these gases produce a pressure of 760 mm Hg at sea level. Each component in the atmosphere does not

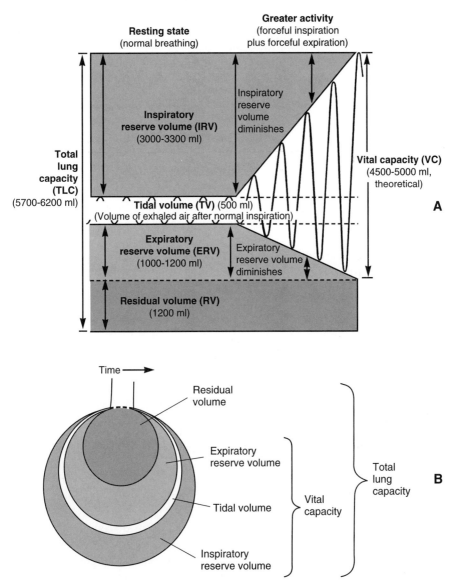

Figure 8-5 Tidal volume. (From Thibodeau GA, Patton KT: *The human body in health and disease,* ed 3, St Louis, 2002, Mosby.)

exert the same amount of pressure. The individual gas pressure is known as *partial pressure.*

2. A gas dissolved in blood also has a partial pressure. The amount of gas capable of dissolving in blood depends on its solubility and partial pressure. Gases always move from higher to lower pressure.[3]

3. The rate at which gases are exchanged depends primarily on the difference between partial pressures. If the gas entering the alveolus has a significantly higher partial pressure than that in the capillary, the gas rapidly

BOX 8-1
Composition of Ambient Air

20.94% oxygen (O_2)
79.02% nitrogen (N_2)
0.04% carbon dioxide (CO_2)

diffuses into the blood. This occurs until the partial pressure in the blood equals that of the alveoli.

a. When N_2O/O_2 is administered, high concentrations of these gases are found in the alveolus, creating a high partial pressure. The capillary, possessing no N_2O originally, is quickly filled.

b. N_2O is not readily absorbed by the blood. Because of this insolubility very little gas is absorbed into blood elements. Within minutes, equilibrium between the partial pressures of the alveolus and capillary is achieved. This quick action continues as the N_2O is carried to the brain; the onset of clinical effect is rapid once the gas reaches the brain.

c. The converse of rapid infusion to the blood is also true. As the N_2O flow is terminated, capillary tension quickly rises to that above alveolar pressure. N_2O is quickly forced into the alveoli and exhaled through the lungs. Trace amounts of N_2O are metabolized in the body; however, the vast majority is removed rapidly through the lungs. During this process, N_2O exits faster than the N_2 that replaces it, thereby diluting the supply of O_2 and reducing the O_2 blood saturation (Sao_2). This phenomenon is called *diffusion hypoxia*.

F. Pulse oximetry provides determination of O_2 saturation of arterial blood. O_2 saturation refers to the amount of O_2 carried by the hemoglobin.

1. In a healthy patient with no pulmonary or cardiovascular disease, O_2 saturation should be between 98% and 100%. There are certain factors that can affect this value. Such factors include altitude (e.g., Denver, Colorado at 5000 feet). Local factors such as nail polish and skin pigmentation can affect the measurement of this value.

2. The pulse oximeter operates on the principle that hemoglobin exists in two forms in the blood, either oxygenated in arterial blood with O_2 molecules loosely bound (HbO_2) or reduced hemoglobin with no O_2 molecules bound (Hb). The amount of arterial saturation (Spo_2) is the ratio of oxygenated hemoglobin to the total. The pulse oximeter measures the absorption of selected wavelengths of light as they pass through living tissue. A sensor is most commonly applied to the fingertip (Figures 8-6 and 8-7). HbO_2 and Hb absorb these wavelengths of light to different extents. The amount of O_2 saturation of arterial blood (Spo_2) as a percentage is displayed on the pulse oximeter screen. Pulse oximeters frequently monitor heart rate as well.

Figure 8-6 Pulse oximeter with digital sensor. (Courtesy Criticare Systems, Inc., Waukesha, Wisconsin.)

Figure 8-7 Digital sensor attached to finger.

3. It is important to recognize that any O_2 saturation level below 90% is a matter of grave concern and is a clear early warning of impending rapid loss of O_2 to the brain.
4. *Although use of a pulse oximeter is not mandated to monitor O_2 saturation for minimal sedation, it is required for moderate sedation according to the ASA Practice Guidelines for Non-anesthesiologists.* Therefore, it can be useful in detecting potential early problems with N_2O/O_2 administration should

the line between minimal and moderate sedation (50% N_2O concentration) be crossed.

G. Diffusion hypoxia.

1. It has been hypothesized that headache, lethargy, and nausea can occur because of decreased O_2 saturation levels in the blood caused by the rapid exit of N_2O upon its termination. The application of 100% pure O_2 for the first 3 to 5 minutes after N_2O termination has been traditionally advocated to prevent O_2 desaturation of blood.

2. Researchers question the clinical significance of diffusion hypoxia and whether these symptoms are even associated. Quarnstrom et al[5] evaluated 104 patients and found no drop in Sao_2. They question the necessity for postoperative O_2. Papageorge, Noonan, and Rosenberg[6] monitored 80 patients and found O_2 decreased with a mean of 2.1%. In this study, all O_2 decreases stabilized independently within 12 seconds to 15 minutes. Dunn-Russell et al[7] assessed 24 children who were allowed to breathe room air after N_2O/O_2 sedation. None exhibited abnormal Sao_2 levels or exhibited any of the associated side effects. Murphy and Splinter[8] claimed the same conclusion with children undergoing general anesthesia. Brodsky et al[9] observed only 3 of 60 patients with Sao_2 decreases. Hovagim et al[10] state that even when postoperative O_2 is given, there may be mild decreases in O_2 saturation.

3. Although researchers claim diffusion hypoxia is not clinically significant, there are patients who experience postoperative headache, lethargy, and nausea. Administering 100% O_2 postoperatively for a minimum of 5 minutes prevents these symptoms from occurring. Lampe et al[11] agree that it continues to be prudent practice to deliver O_2 postoperatively. We concur that it is useful and should always be employed.

VI. Management of Patients Experiencing Moderate Sedation (Levels of N_2O above 50%)

A. Guidelines. Nonanesthesiologists who treat patients in a hospital setting are legally required to adhere to the ASA practice guidelines previously referenced. Private practitioners, although not required to follow these guidelines, should seriously consider using these standards in their offices because the guidelines describe the standards of care that have been established by the practitioners' hospital-based peers. Again, the practitioner is responsible for the possible complications associated with the intended level of sedation and those associated with the next (deeper) level. Therefore because moderate sedation may occur or be intended, considerations for obstructed airway and preprocedure fasting guidelines are addressed.

B. Airway obstruction in the upper airway represents an acute life-threatening situation.[12]

1. This is commonly the result of the dorsum of the tongue occluding with the posterior pharyngeal wall. Another common cause of airway obstruction is the presence of a foreign body.[13]

2. During moderate sedation, the laryngeal and pharyngeal reflexes should remain intact at all times, thereby allowing the cough and gag reflexes to protect the airway.

C. The universal distress signal for choking is to grasp the throat with both hands.

1. If a foreign body airway obstruction is suspected in a conscious individual, ask the person "Are you choking?"

2. Apply the Heimlich maneuver until the foreign object is expelled or the person becomes unconscious.

3. Summon emergency personnel immediately for any unconscious person. Perform chest thrusts and attempt to ventilate the lungs similar to cardiopulmonary resuscitation (CPR) until medical assistance arrives.[14]

D. A simple hyperextension (head tilt–chin lift) or jaw thrust maneuver should relieve an airway obstruction that is not caused by the presence of a foreign body.

1. A partial airway obstruction will allow the patient to make sounds. A snoring sound can indicate a partial airway obstruction caused by the posterior displacement of the tongue.[13]

2. There is no sound with a complete airway obstruction.

3. An airway obstruction caused by oversedation from N_2O/O_2 administration can be quickly reversed with the termination of the N_2O and the administration of 100% O_2. Note that a full face mask replacing the nasal hood and a reservoir bag filled with oxygen can provide positive pressurized oxygen into the lungs.

E. The pulse oximeter should be left in place at all times to continuously monitor oxygen saturation.

F. Aspiration of vomitus is unlikely when the protective airway reflexes are intact.

1. Should vomiting occur, the patient should be placed in the Trendelenburg position on the right side to keep the vomitus in the mouth.

2. The pharynx should be suctioned to remove any vomitus. O_2 should be administered and the patient should be evaluated for the possibility of any aspiration.[13]

G. Preprocedure fasting guidelines are recommended in the ASA practice guidelines. These guidelines are to be used when moderate sedation is achieved intentionally or unintentionally. It is recommended that a light meal with no fried or fatty foods be consumed at least 6 hours before sedation procedures and that no liquids be consumed within 2 hours of the procedure. A complete summary of the ASA preprocedure fasting guidelines may be found in Chapter 10.

REFERENCES

1. Light RW: Mechanics of respiration. In George RB et al, editors: *Chest medicine: essentials of pulmonary and critical care medicine*, Baltimore, 1995, Williams & Wilkins.

2. George RB, Chesson AL, Rennard SI: Functional anatomy of the respiratory system. In George RB et al, editors: *Chest medicine: essentials of pulmonary and critical care medicine*, Baltimore, 1995, Williams & Wilkins.

3. Stoelting RD: *Pharmacology and physiology in anesthetic practice,* ed 2, Philadelphia, 1991, JB Lippincott.
4. Shapiro BA: *Oxygenation: measurement and clinical assessment,* Philadelphia, 1979, JB Lippincott.
5. Quarnstrom FC et al: Clinical study of diffusion hypoxia after nitrous oxide analgesia, *Anesth Prog* 38:21, 1991.
6. Papageorge MB, Noonan LW Jr, Rosenberg M: Diffusion hypoxia: another view, *Anesth Pain Control Dent* 2:143, 1993.
7. Dunn-Russell T et al: Oxygen saturation and diffusion hypoxia in children following nitrous oxide sedation, *Pediatr Dent* 16:88, 1993.
8. Murphy IL, Splinter WM: The clinical significance of diffusion hypoxia in children, *Can J Anaesth* 37:S40, 1990.
9. Brodsky JB et al: Diffusion hypoxia: a reappraisal using pulse oximetry, *J Clin Mon* 4:244, 1988.
10. Hovagim AR et al: Arterial oxygen desaturation in adult dental patients receiving conscious sedation, *J Oral Maxillofac Surg* 47:936, 1989.
11. Lampe GH et al: Postoperative hypoxemia after nonabdominal surgery: a frequent event not caused by nitrous oxide, *Anesth Analg* 71:597, 1990.
12. Malamed SF: Medical emergencies in the dental office, ed 5, St Louis, 2000, Mosby.
13. Malamed SF: Sedation: a guide to patient management, ed 4, St Louis, 2003, Mosby.
14. American Heart Association: Guidelines 2000 for CPR and emergency cardiovascular care, *Curr Emerg Cardiovasc Care* 11(3):11, 2000.

SUGGESTED READINGS

Artru AA: Survival time during hypoxia: effects of nitrous oxide, thiopental, and hypothermia, *Anesth Analg* 67:913, 1988.
Eger EI II: Respiratory effects of nitrous oxide. In Eger EI II: *Nitrous oxide N$_2$O,* New York, 1985, Elsevier Science Publishing.
Mueller WA et al: Pulse oximetry monitoring of sedated pediatric dental patients, *Anesth Prog* 32:237, 1985.
Papageorge MB et al: Supplemental oxygen after outpatient oral and maxillofacial surgery, *Anesth Prog* 39:24, 1993.

9

N₂O and its Interaction with the Body

The scientific study of N_2O and its effect on the human body began with Horace Wells and has continued since that time. The literature is deluged with articles covering virtually every possible aspect of the drug. N_2O is an inhalant anesthetic drug, and its interaction with the body is compared with that of other inhalation anesthetics such as halothane, isoflurane, and enflurane. The debate as to whether N_2O is a friend or foe to the human body has been interesting to follow. Dr. Edmond Eger II, one of the most notable experts in the world on the subject, has had varying opinions on the virtues of N_2O. However, in a recent study Eger et al[1] examined several controversial aspects of the effects of N_2O and concluded that continued use of N_2O should be supported. Healthcare professionals should always encourage further scientific questioning and study.

I. N₂O Interaction with Body Systems and Conditions

A. Cardiovascular system
1. N_2O does not negatively affect the cardiovascular system to produce any significant physiologic changes. The interaction of several cardiovascular functions such as contractility, output, stroke volume, heart rate, and arrhythmias with N_2O have been researched in the past.[1-5] Overall, N_2O has proven to be slightly cardiotonic.
2. N_2O effects on cardiac output differ in the literature. Slight increases have been noted as well as mild decreases. Dosage and the sympathomimetic effects of the drug may account for subtle differences.[1-5]
3. Blood flow to major organs is not significantly affected.[3]
4. N_2O with O_2 does not create adverse cardiovascular conditions. Conversely, it has a positive effect on myocardial ischemia by providing supplemental O_2 and can be very helpful in myocardial infarction.[6,7]
5. Blood pressure effects from N_2O may be dose related. In most instances blood pressure is not affected by the N_2O concentrations commonly used in ambulatory settings. Eger et al[1] found blood pressure readings to be lowered when N_2O/O_2 was used. This potential decrease in blood pressure is a result of relaxation because N_2O does not have any direct effect on the myocardium or voluntary skeletal muscle.

6. N_2O/O_2 sedation does not pose any significant negative effect on the cardiovascular system and can therefore be used with common conditions such as the following:
   a. Atherosclerosis or arteriosclerosis
   b. Rheumatic fever, heart murmur, congenital conditions
   c. Angina pectoris, myocardial infarction
   d. Surgery (valve, pacemaker, bypass, transplant)
   e. Hypertension
   f. All bleeding diatheses
B. Central nervous system (CNS)
   1. N_2O, like other anesthetics, has the ability to depress the CNS; however, the exact mechanism is unknown.[4]
   2. Comparatively, N_2O's effect on cerebral blood flow, intracranial pressure, and O_2 consumption appears to be less significant than that of other inhaled anesthetics.[4,8]
   3. The dosage of N_2O has an effect on the frequency and voltage changes on electroencephalograms (EEGs).[4,8]
   4. Because of the rapid replacement of N_2 with N_2O in air spaces, notable intracranial pressure increases were found in cases of pneumoencephalography. N_2O should not be used for 1 week after this procedure.[8]
   5. Evidence of injury to the nervous system has been shown in cases of *chronic* exposure to N_2O. Numbness and weakness in the extremities are seen as symptoms, as is ataxic gait.[2] This subject is discussed in detail in Chapter 17.
   6. N_2O/O_2 sedation does not pose any significant negative effect on the CNS, and therefore can be used with common conditions such as:
      a. Cerebrovascular accident (stroke)
      b. Seizure disorder, fainting spells
      c. Parkinson's disease, etc.
C. Respiratory system
   1. Upper respiratory tract infections or conditions commonly compromise air exchange through the nose. If the patient is unable to breathe through the nose, insufficient amounts of N_2O/O_2 will enter the respiratory system.
      a. Any type of common infection leading to a cold, cough, sinus infection, bronchitis, allergy-related symptoms, etc. may occlude the nasal passages such that adequate air exchange at the alveolar level will be incomplete.
      b. Additionally, if N_2O/O_2 is used for an individual with mild symptoms, the drying effect of the gases may create mucous plugs and negatively affect the pulmonary tree. Again, sedation may be incomplete and inadequate.
      c. Sinus cavities represent rigid, noncompliant air spaces. The nonexpansive nature of these areas leads to an increase in pressure when N_2O is administered. When sinusitis is present, the additional pressure may be uncomfortable for the patient.

2. Although rare, silent regurgitation and subsequent aspiration need to be considered with N_2O/O_2 sedation. The concern lies in whether pharyngeal-laryngeal reflexes remain intact. This problem can be avoided by not allowing a patient to go into an unconscious state.[9]

   a. Dye studies done with a 5- to 10-minute exposure to 50% N_2O were negative for aspiration[10]; no evidence of aspiration occurred in 25 children given N_2O concentrations between 20% and 65%.[11]

   b. Most procedures performed in an ambulatory health setting are time intensive, and patients may not have fasted. Therefore, the potential for positive aspiration resulting from silent regurgitation does exist.

   c. Because this is a potentially life-threatening situation, it is important to use the appropriate *titration* technique when administering N_2O/O_2 sedation to avoid oversedation. Continuous monitoring of the patient should always be carried out.

3. Patients susceptible to hypoxia because of airway resistance, impaired function, or movement appear to be at a slight risk from N_2O/O_2 sedation but not more than any other substances. Eger[9] indicates that this may not be a significant issue.

   a. Examples of conditions in this category are emphysema, chronic bronchitis, and asthma. *There has never been a reported allergy to N_2O.* Its use is not contraindicated for asthma patients because it is nonirritating to mucous membranes. In fact, the sedative nature of N_2O/O_2 has a positive influence on asthmatic patients because anxiety can trigger an asthmatic episode.

   b. For patients chronically debilitated with other respiratory conditions, N_2O/O_2 may be considered relatively contraindicated (Box 9-1).

     i. Some of these patients may be on hypoxic drive. Although CO_2 normally initiates respiration in healthy individuals, O_2 may be the stimulus for those compromised with chronic obstructive pulmonary diseases (COPD).

     ii. Patients with severe chronic respiratory diseases should receive medical consultation before undergoing any type of sedation. Any type of sedation may risk further depression of their respiratory drive.

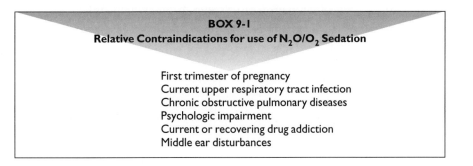

BOX 9-1

Relative Contraindications for use of N_2O/O_2 Sedation

First trimester of pregnancy
Current upper respiratory tract infection
Chronic obstructive pulmonary diseases
Psychologic impairment
Current or recovering drug addiction
Middle ear disturbances

    iii. In the majority of cases, persons on hypoxic drive are very ill. Some will not be able to be treated in an ambulatory setting; most represent an ASA III or IV classification (see Chapter 10). Medical consultation is recommended before any treatment.

4. Patients with cystic fibrosis may incur bullae as a complication of this disease, again because of the expansive nature of the gas. N_2O would be contraindicated in this case.

5. The condition of pneumothorax (air or gas in the pleural cavity) may be complicated with N_2O. The expansive quality of the gas causes increased expansion of the size of the pneumothorax. This condition demands medical attention. In general anesthesia, if 75% N_2O is delivered, the volume of the space can be increased up to 300%.[12] Although in the ambulatory setting the doses of N_2O are much smaller, the pharmacodynamic nature of the gas is constant. N_2O/O_2 sedation should be avoided in this situation.

6. Therefore N_2O/O_2 sedation presents the following recommendations regarding the respiratory system:
   a. Emphysema—physician discretion for hypoxic drive
   b. Chronic bronchitis—physician discretion for hypoxic drive
   c. Tuberculosis—sterilize contaminated items
   d. Human immunodeficiency virus/acquired immune deficiency syndrome (HIV/AIDS)—sterilize contaminated items
   e. Upper respiratory tract infections—postpone N_2O/O_2 until resolved
   f. Pneumothorax—postpone N_2O/O_2 until resolved
   g. Cystic fibrosis—postpone N_2O/O_2 until resolved

D. Hematopoietic system
   1. Megaloblastic bone marrow changes have been found in patients who have been exposed to high concentrations of N_2O for an extended period.[13] N_2O has been implicated in the interference of the vitamin B_{12}-dependent enzyme methionine synthase. This enzyme is necessary for DNA synthesis and erythrocyte production.[4,8]
   2. Another concern with hematopoietic conditions is the decrease in O_2 available to the body because of red blood cell deficiency, impairment, destruction, and/or other conditions affecting red blood cells. Inhalation sedation is often recommended because of the supplemental O_2 it delivers.[14]
   3. Therefore N_2O/O_2 sedation can be administered for the following:
      a. Anemias
      b. Methemoglobinemia
      c. Sickle cell anemia
      d. Leukemia
      e. Hemophilia
      f. Polycythemia vera

E. Endocrine system
   1. Inhalation sedation using N_2O/O_2 has *no* negative effect on the endocrine system.

2. Therefore it poses no risk for individuals with any condition involving this system, such as the following:
    a. Diabetes
    b. Thyroid gland dysfunction
    c. Adrenal dysfunction
F. Hepatic system
    1. N$_2$O is *not* metabolized in the liver, nor does it affect the liver in the presence of liver impairment.[1,15-17]
    2. Therefore N$_2$O/O$_2$ sedation does not pose any effect on the following conditions:
        a. Hepatitis
        b. Jaundice
        c. Cirrhosis
G. Gastrointestinal system
    1. Because of the expansive nature of the gas and its propensity for insufflating air spaces within the body, N$_2$O diffuses into these areas much more rapidly than N$_2$ exits. The gas entering nonrigid-walled air spaces in the body causes the spaces to expand. This expansion and possible pressure can be problematic.
    2. The bowel exemplifies a nonrigid air space in which expansion occurs. If a patient has a bowel obstruction, it is less desirable to use N$_2$O/O$_2$ sedation because the N$_2$O can affect the condition by increasing expansion, pressure, and discomfort.[18]
    3. Therefore the following recommendations regarding the gastrointestinal system and N$_2$O/O$_2$ sedation are made:
        a. Ulcer—no negative effect using N$_2$O/O$_2$
        b. Obstructions—postpone N$_2$O/O$_2$ until resolved
H. Genitourinary and reproductive systems
    1. N$_2$O/O$_2$ sedation does not pose any negative effect on the genitourinary system itself. Any time disease transmissibility is an issue, proper infection control procedures and sterilization of appropriate equipment are recommended.
    2. Pregnancy is a normal physiologic state that requires twice the demand for folate. Treatment considerations are important during organogenesis in the first trimester and when low O$_2$-tension levels are possible in the last trimester. Most pharmacologic agents cross the placental barrier; N$_2$O is no exception.
        a. It is necessary to maintain adequate O$_2$ levels to prevent spontaneous abortion. However, the O$_2$ fail-safe feature incorporated in updated equipment prevents this occurrence.
        b. The N$_2$O/O$_2$ combination has been a commonly used pharmacologic agent in obstetrics. Research confirms its safety with pregnant women.[19] In case of pregnancy, the following items regarding N$_2$O/O$_2$ sedation in the ambulatory setting should be considered:
            i. Obtain appropriate medical consultation before the use of any drug for the duration of the pregnancy.

    ii. Avoid N_2O during the first trimester. N_2O, when delivered appropriately, should not physiologically threaten the fetus; however, like radiation, N_2O/O_2 could be blamed unfairly should fetal anomalies occur.

    iii. It is best to leave the decision whether to use N_2O/O_2 sedation to the patient and attending medical personnel.

  3. Therefore regarding these body systems, recommendations for N_2O/O_2 sedation are as follows:

    a. Kidney disease—no negative effect using N_2O/O_2

    b. Sexually transmitted diseases—sterilize contaminated items

    c. Pregnancy—medical consultation recommended

I. Neuromuscular system

  1. N_2O does not provide direct skeletal muscle relaxation. In high concentrations, muscle rigidity can be seen with N_2O secondary to anxiety.[20]

  2. N_2O/O_2 has no effect on patients with neuromuscular conditions.

  3. Therefore the use of N_2O/O_2 sedation can be recommended with the following conditions involving the neuromuscular system:

    a. Multiple sclerosis

    b. Muscular dystrophy

    c. Cerebral palsy

    d. Myasthenia gravis

    e. Other

J. Sensory systems

  1. Middle ear disturbances

    a. Because N_2O infiltrates the rigid, noncompliant area of the middle ear, increased pressure results. Complications have been noted with middle ear surgical procedures using N_2O.[21] Significant damage such as tympanic membrane rupture, graft displacement, and other complications have been observed.[21-26] Also, the negative pressure that results from the rapid departure of N_2O after general anesthesia can cause other side effects, especially after recent ear, nose, and throat complications.[27]

    b. The conditions listed above refer to surgical procedures using anesthetic concentrations of N_2O. There is no mention if these complications occur with lower concentrations used in minimal sedation. Therefore medical consultation is advised and N_2O/O_2 sedation used or postponed upon recommendation by the physician in the following situations:

      i. Middle ear conditions (i.e., infections, grafts, etc.)—medical consultation advised

      ii. Recent ear, nose, throat infections—medical consultation advised

  2. Eye surgery

    a. A safety alert was published about patients and recent ophthalmic surgery in which perfluoropropane or sulfur hexafluoride gas was used. In these patients there is a "gas bubble" in the eye that is normal to the healing process that could expand with N_2O and complicate healing or promote injury.[28]

    b. Patients should be questioned about recent ophthalmic surgery before using N_2O/O_2 sedation.

K. Cancer
1. N_2O does not combine with any of the formed blood elements, nor does it affect metastatic cells.[14]
2. N_2O/O_2 has been used in the final stages of life as an adjuvant to other pharmacologic methods for pain and anxiety management. In these situations the untoward effects caused by chronic exposure to N_2O are irrelevant.[29,30]
3. Therefore N_2O/O_2 sedation can provide additional comfort for the following condition:
    a. Cancer—positive analgesic effect in final stages of life

L. Mind-altering conditions
1. Mind-altering conditions must be carefully considered before N_2O/O_2 administration.
2. If patients are unable to understand the procedure and its effects, they may negatively perceive the associated signs and symptoms of N_2O/O_2 sedation.
3. If the patient is suffering or recovering from addiction or mental illness, the relaxing, euphoric sensations may exacerbate or trigger unwanted episodes or encourage addictive behaviors. Discretion is warranted.
4. Therefore careful consideration should be taken regarding N_2O/O_2 sedation when the following conditions exist:
    a. Mental illness
    b. Mental retardation
    c. Autism
    d. Alzheimer's disease
    e. Chemical dependency, including alcoholism and substance abuse

M. Allergies
1. For more than 150 years there have been no known reported allergies to N_2O.
2. Therefore, N_2O/O_2 sedation does not pose any effect on any type of allergy.
3. Persons sensitive to latex may experience contact dermatitis when using the nasal hood. Latex-free nasal hoods are available from each equipment manufacturer in the United States.

N. Malignant hyperthermia (MH)
1. This condition may unexpectedly occur as a result of an individual's response to certain drugs. Patients who know of familial tendencies and history can be tested to avoid this problem.
2. N_2O/O_2 sedation is not considered a trigger for malignant hyperthermia and can be safely administered to MH-susceptible individuals.

O. Nutritional disorders
1. N_2O/O_2 sedation does not affect any nutritional condition.

II. N₂O Interaction with Medications

A. There is no direct interaction of N_2O with medications taken by the patient.[31]

B. N_2O can have a synergistic effect with certain other drugs (i.e., sedative-hypnotics).

C. N_2O may enhance drugs that are used directly to induce sleep or that list drowsiness as a side effect.

D. Patients currently using bleomycin sulfate, an antineoplastic agent used typically for the treatment of lymphomas, testicular tumors, and squamous cell carcinomas, can increase the incidence of pulmonary fibrosis and other pulmonary disease. This occurs only indirectly if O_2 is administered concomitantly with N_2O in concentrations over 30%. Although this is an unusual situation, it must be regarded.[32]

III. Additional Considerations Regarding N₂O/O₂ Use

A. Altered mental states or levels of consciousness indicate a situation warranting careful consideration before N_2O/O_2 administration.

1. N_2O/O_2 use should be avoided for a patient intoxicated with drugs or alcohol. Alcohol and barbiturates are CNS depressants.

   a. Although alcohol is initially a stimulant, it has been historically prescribed and acknowledged as a mild anxiolytic over time. It should never be present when a healthcare provider is administering N_2O and O_2.

   b. Barbiturates are quite effective sedative agents when prescribed in a professional manner; however, patients prescribing their own drugs and dosages before their appointments should not be treated in these settings.

2. Patients under psychiatric and/or psychologic care should be carefully considered before N_2O/O_2 use. Many patients are treated with antidepressant or other psychotropic drugs. Drug interaction is not at issue in these cases, but rather the potential for exacerbating the negative aspects of the condition. Seek medical consultation before N_2O/O_2 administration.

3. For those professionals in emergency medicine, whether in the field or hospital, it is unwise to use N_2O/O_2 for anyone in shock, in a semiconscious state, or with head or facial injuries.

4. Severely phobic individuals will not benefit by N_2O/O_2 administration. These persons should be in the care of a competent expert in behavior management. It is unlikely that N_2O/O_2 will be able to provide adequate relief to accomplish the intended procedure. It is likely that N_2O/O_2 will make the situation worse because the patient will resist the calming effects of the drug. Physical agitation and acts of aggression can result. Deep sedation or general anesthesia will, most likely, be the procedure of choice in this situation.

5. In some cases, patients with claustrophobic tendencies may feel uncomfortable using a nasal hood. Often these patients relax sufficiently during N$_2$O/O$_2$ sedation that this is not a problem.

B. When time is taken to explain the N$_2$O/O$_2$ procedure and words are carefully chosen to present the positive effects, most patients will consent. If a patient is unwilling or does not give consent, the practitioner must never force the continuance of the procedure. This may destroy any patient-operator trust and place the practitioner in legal jeopardy.

REFERENCES

1. Eger EI, II, et al: Clinical pharmacology of nitrous oxide: an argument for its continued use, *Anesth Anal* 71:575, 1990.
2. Eger EI, II, Gaskey NJ: A review of the present status of nitrous oxide, *J Assoc Nurse Anes* 54:29, 1986.
3. Eisele JH, Jr: Cardiovascular effects of nitrous oxide. In Eger EI II: *Nitrous oxide N$_2$O*, New York, 1985, Elsevier Science Publishing.
4. Stoelting RK: *Pharmacology and physiology in anesthetic practice*, ed 2, Philadelphia, 1991, JB Lippincott.
5. Stoelting RK, Miller RD: *Basics of anesthesia*, ed 2, New York, 1989, Churchill Livingstone.
6. Thompson PL, Lown B: Nitrous oxide as an analgesic in acute myocardial infarction, *J Am Med Assoc* 235:924, 1976.
7. Kerr F et al: Nitrous oxide analgesia in myocardial infarction, *Lancet* 1:63, 1972.
8. Frost EA: Central nervous system effects of nitrous oxide. In Eger EI II: *Nitrous oxide N$_2$O*, New York, 1985, Elsevier Science Publishing.
9. Eger EI, II: Respiratory effects of nitrous oxide. In Eger EI II: *Nitrous oxide N$_2$O*, New York, 1985, Elsevier Science Publishing.
10. Cleaton-Jones P: The laryngeal-closure reflex and nitrous oxide-oxygen anesthesia, *Anesthesiology* 45:569, 1976.
11. Roberts GJ, Wignall BK: Efficacy of the laryngeal reflex during oxygen-nitrous oxide sedation (relative analgesia), *Br J Anesth* 54:1277, 1982.
12. Eger EI II, Saidman LJ: Hazards of nitrous oxide anesthesia in bowel obstruction and pneumothorax, *Anesthesiology* 26:61, 1965.
13. Nunn JE: Clinical aspects of the interaction between nitrous oxide and vitamin B$_{12}$, *Br J Anesth* 59:3, 1987.
14. Malamed SF: *Sedation: a guide to patient management*, ed 4, St Louis, 2003, Mosby.
15. Brodsky JB: Toxicity of nitrous oxide. In Eger EI II: *Nitrous oxide N$_2$O*, New York, 1985, Elsevier Science Publishing.
16. Lampe GJ et al: Nitrous oxide does not impair hepatic function on young or old surgical patients, *Anesth Analg* 71:606, 1990.
17. Longnecker DE, Miller FL: Pharmacology of inhalation anesthetics. In Rogers M et al, editors: *Principles and practice of anesthesiology*, St Louis, 1993, Mosby.
18. Eger EI II: Pharmacokinetics. In Eger EI II, editor: *Nitrous oxide N$_2$O*, New York, 1985, Elsevier Science Publishing.
19. Marx FG, Bassell GM: Nitrous oxide in obstetrics. In Eger EI II: *Nitrous oxide N$_2$O*, New York, 1985, Elsevier Science Publishing.
20. Miller RD: Neuromuscular effects of nitrous oxide. In Eger EI II: *Nitrous oxide N$_2$O*, New York, 1985, Elsevier Science Publishing.
21. Munson ES: Complications of nitrous oxide anesthesia for ear surgery, *Anesthesiology* 11(3):559, 1993.

22. Donlon JV, Jr: Anesthesia and eye, ear, nose, and throat surgery. In Miller RD: *Anesthesia*, ed 4, New York, 1994, Churchill Livingstone.

23. Barash P, Cullen B, Stoelting R: *Clinical anesthesia*, ed 2, Philadelphia, 1992, JB Lippincott.

24. Mann MS, Woodsford PV, Jones RM: Anesthetic carrier gases, *Anesthesiology* 40:8, 1985.

25. Waun JE, Sweitzer RH, Hamilton WK: Effect of nitrous oxide on middle ear mechanics and hearing activity, *Anesthesiology* 28:846, 1967.

26. Ohryn M: Tympanic membrane rupture following general anesthesia with nitrous oxide: a case report, *J Am Assoc Nurse Anesth* 63:42, 1995.

27. Chinn K et al: Middle ear pressure variation: effect of nitrous oxide, *Laryngoscope* 107(3):357, 1997.

28. Berthold M: Safety alert: nitrous oxide–screen for recent ophthalmic surgery, *ADA News* 6:20, 2002.

29. Fosburg MT, Crone RK: Nitrous oxide analgesia for refractory pain in the terminally ill, *J Am Med Assoc* 250:511, 1983.

30. Foley LM: The treatment of pain in the patient with cancer, *CA Cancer J Clin* 36:194, 1986.

31. Dale O, Brown BR, Jr: Clinical pharmacokinetics of the inhalational anaesthetics, *Clin Pharmacokinet* 12:145, 1987.

32. *Physician's desk reference*, ed 55, Montvale, NJ, 2001, Medical Economics.

10

Patient Assessment

To best serve a patient it is imperative that the healthcare provider obtain an initial medical history from the patient. This information is acquired through a formal interview and updated at each visit. Undivided attention is necessary to assess the patient's physiologic and psychologic status so that the best pain and anxiety management option may be selected. The ASA Task Force[1] agrees that obtaining a preprocedure evaluation increases the likelihood of success during sedation and decreases the chance for adverse outcomes. Even friends and relatives whom practitioners think they know well must have this formal scrutiny. Hence the familiar axiom: *Never treat a stranger.*

I. Obtaining Patient History Information

A. The patient often completes questions about health and personal information in the reception area, with no further inquiries made by a practitioner. It is assumed that this information is seen before patient treatment; however, this may not always be the case.

B. It is advantageous to obtain this information through direct interaction with patients. Information exchanged through a formal interview enables professionals to further question responses and make an assessment of patient pain and anxiety. The person directly involved with the treatment of the patient should complete the interview.

C. Information specific to sedation that should be collected includes: (1) abnormalities of the major organ systems, (2) previous adverse experience with sedation or analgesia, (3) drug allergies, current medications, and potential drug interactions, (4) time and nature of last oral intake, and (5) history of tobacco, alcohol, or substance use or abuse.[1]

D. It is highly recommended to include a question(s) about pain and anxiety on the health history form itself.[2] This provides patients with a nonthreatening way to communicate anxious feelings that they may be hesitant to divulge verbally. Examples of such questions include "Is there anything about being here for treatment that bothers you?" "Have you had a negative experience in an office or clinic before?" or "Have you previously required special procedures or medication for nervousness before an appointment?"

   1. Scales indicating pain and/or anxiety levels can be included on the health history form as well.

2. Some patients will feel comfortable about communicating their anxious feelings verbally. Others will not admit to uncomfortable feelings but may show outward signs such as sweating, shaking, syncope, etc. In either case, those initial minutes of dialogue are valuable for gathering information.

E. A professional can then use the health information obtained from the interview to make an assessment about the health risk to the patient before performing a medical or dental procedure.

II. Assessment of Patient Risk

A. The American Society of Anesthesiologists (ASA) developed a method of classifying patients according to medical risk. The Physical Status Classification system was initiated in the early 1960s and is recognized around the world.[3] Its applicability and validity for almost every health discipline is the reason for its continued use today. During assessment of the health and physical status of patients, this system helps determine if a patient is an appropriate candidate for sedation (Box 10-1).

B. The ASA Physical Status Classification system.[4]

1. ASA I—Patients with no systemic disease. These patients are able to tolerate mild physical exertion and psychologic stresses. They do not possess any organic, physiologic, biochemical, or psychiatric disturbances. This patient may be considered an appropriate candidate for N_2O/O_2 sedation.

2. ASA II—Patients with mild-to-moderate physiologic disturbance that is under good control. There is no significant compromise of normal activity; however, the patient's specific condition could possibly affect the safety of surgery and anesthesia. Depending on their particular situation, these patients are usually considered appropriate candidates for N_2O/O_2 sedation.

3. ASA III—Patients with a major systemic disturbance that is difficult to control. There is significant compromise of normal activity for this patient. This situation creates a significant impact on surgery and anesthesia. Medical consultation is recommended for these patients. These patients present greater risk for treatment; however, N_2O/O_2 sedation may still be used following medical advice.

4. ASA IV—Patients with severe and potentially life-threatening systemic disease that significantly limits their activity are not usually seen in an ambulatory health setting. Because of their unstable health problems, they are categorized as high risk for many situations; the potential for an acute emergency situation is great. Seek medical consultation and/or referral. N_2O/O_2 is usually not indicated except in emergency situations.

5. ASA V—Moribund patients in whom immediate surgery is the last effort to save their lives. In some cases N_2O/O_2 is recommended for pain and anxiety relief in these final stages.

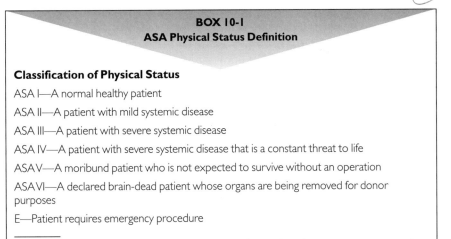

BOX 10-1
ASA Physical Status Definition

Classification of Physical Status

ASA I—A normal healthy patient

ASA II—A patient with mild systemic disease

ASA III—A patient with severe systemic disease

ASA IV—A patient with severe systemic disease that is a constant threat to life

ASA V—A moribund patient who is not expected to survive without an operation

ASA VI—A declared brain-dead patient whose organs are being removed for donor purposes

E—Patient requires emergency procedure

From the American Society of Anesthesiologists: *Manual for anesthesia department organization and management,* Park Ridge, IL, 2003, American Society of Anesthesiologists. Reprinted with permission of the American Society of Anesthesiologists, Park Ridge, Illinois.

6. ASA VI—The patient in this classification is clinically dead but being maintained for organ donation.
7. ASA E—Desination for a patient in any ASA classification requiring an emergency procedure.

III. Preprocedural Patient Evaluation

A. Vital signs
   1. Evaluating preoperative, intraoperative, and postoperative vital signs is considered the standard of care by the ASA, ADSA, and several other professional health societies and organizations.[5] Vital sign values should be recorded in the patient's chart each time they are measured. It is appropriate to obtain baseline values at the initial visit and then periodically thereafter.
   2. Depending on the discipline, specialties with established guidelines for delivering anesthesia and sedation may recommend that vital signs be measured whenever N_2O/O_2 is used.[6-8] State governing bodies may also require that vital signs be measured.[9]
   3. There are a total of six vital signs: height, weight, body temperature, blood pressure, pulse, and respiration.
   4. Depending on the clinical setting and treatment being performed, some vital signs are measured more frequently than others. Blood pressure, pulse, and respiration are the most dynamic vital signs and should be recorded at each visit. Oxygen saturation level and a pain score have been advocated in some cases to be included with vital sign information.[10]
   5. Vital sign measurements recommended for minimal sedation are blood pressure, pulse, and respiration. These should be obtained preoperatively to provide a baseline reference before N_2O/O_2 administration.

Postoperative vital signs serve as a measure of recovery from N_2O/O_2 sedation. These values are compared with those obtained preoperatively and are assessed for the degree of variation. Details about recovery from N_2O/O_2 sedation are found in Chapter 14.

B. Auscultation of the heart and lungs and evaluation of the airway are recommended by the ASA Task Force before sedation.

1. A precordial-pretracheal stethoscope is a device used to monitor respiration and heart sounds. The stethoscope head is weighted and can be secured in place with tape. The tubing connects to one or two earpieces. The pretracheal scope head is placed in the midline of the neck near the lower end of the trachea. At this location, sounds of air exchange can easily be heard. The scope can also be placed in the precordial region over the heart. At this location, both heart and lung sounds can be heard[11] (Figure 10-1).

2. Preprocedure evaluation of the airway can uncover airway abnormalities that could increase the likelihood of airway obstruction.[1] The evaluation includes questioning the patient about previous problems with anesthesia or sedation, sleep problems, advanced rheumatoid arthritis, or chromosomal abnormalities. Physical evaluation includes the determination of size and limitations of the head, neck, and mouth, as well as variations in occlusion and teeth (Box 10-2).

3. Remember, the operator must be prepared to manage the complications associated with the next (deeper) level of sedation beyond that which is intended.[1]

IV. Patient Preparation

A. Because sedation affects airway reflexes proportional to the level of sedation, it is suggested that preprocedure fasting can decrease the risk of aspiration of stomach contents should the patient vomit.[1]

1. Patients who are using N_2O/O_2 for elective procedures should not drink fluids or eat solid foods for a sufficient time before the procedure to allow for gastric emptying (Box 10-3).[1]

2. Although vomiting should not occur during minimal sedation, it is necessary to be prepared for the adverse conditions that are associated with moderate sedation.

B. Before N_2O/O_2 sedation the patient should be informed about the intent of the procedure and how it will be accomplished along with the risks, benefits, and alternatives to its use.[1,9]

1. Informed consent should be obtained from competent patients and/or legal guardians of children or others each time N_2O/O_2 is administered.

2. Although the law does not mandate written consent, it is advisable to have a specific form with the information followed by the patient's or guardian's signature and the date. An example of a consent form appropriate for N_2O/O_2 administration can be found in Appendix D. An overview of the Health Insurance Portability and Accoutability Act of 1996 (HIPAA) can be found in Appendix F.

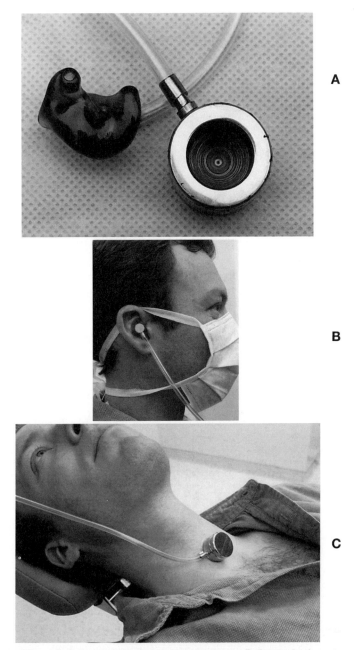

Figure 10-1   A, Pretracheal stethoscope and earpiece. **B,** Pretracheal earpiece placement. **C,** Pretracheal stethoscope placement. (From Malamed SF: *Sedation: a guide to patient management,* ed 4, St Louis, 2003, Mosby.)

BOX 10-2
Airway Assessment Procedures for Sedation and Analgesia

Positive-pressure ventilation, with or without tracheal intubation, may be necessary if respiratory compromise develops during sedation-analgesia. This may be difficult in patients with atypical airway anatomy. In addition, some airway abnormalities may increase the likelihood of airway obstruction during spontaneous ventilation. Some factors that may be associated with difficulty in airway management are the following:

History
Previous problems with anesthesia or sedation
Stridor, snoring, or sleep apnea
Advanced rheumatoid arthritis
Chromosomal abnormality (e.g., trisomy 21)

Physical Examination
Habitus
Significant obesity (especially involving the neck and facial structures)

Head and neck
Short neck, limited neck extension, decreased hyoid-mental distance (<3 cm in an adult), neck mass, cervical spine disease or trauma, tracheal deviation, dysmorphic facial features (e.g., Pierre-Robin syndrome)

Mouth
Small opening (<3 cm in an adult), edentulous, protruding incisors, loose or capped teeth, dental appliances, high arched palate, macroglossia, tonsillar hypertrophy, nonvisible uvula

Jaw
Micrognathia, retrognathia, trismus, significant malocclusion

---

Modified from ASA Task Force: Practice guidelines for sedation and analgesia by non-anesthesiologists, *Anesthesiology* 96(4):1004, 2002. Reprinted with permission of the American Society of Anesthesiologists, Park Ridge, Illinois.

BOX 10-3
Preprocedure Fasting Guidelines

Ingested Material	Minimum Fasting Period
Clear liquid	2 hours
Nonhuman milk	6 hours
Light meals	6 hours

These recommendations apply to healthy patients who are undergoing elective procedures. They are not intended for women in labor. Following the guidelines does not guarantee complete gastric emptying has occurred.
The fasting periods apply to all ages.
Examples of clear liquids include water, fruit juices without pulp, carbonated beverages, clear tea, and black coffee.
Because nonhuman milk is similar to solids in gastric emptying time, the amount ingested must be considered when determining an appropriate fasting period.
A light meal typically consists of toast and clear liquids. Meals that include fried or fatty foods or meat may prolong gastric emptying time. Both the amount and type of food ingested must be considered when determining an appropriate fasting period.

Modified from ASA Task Force: Practice guidelines for sedation and analgesia by non-anesthesiologists, *Anesthesiology* 96(4):1004, 2002. Reprinted with permission of the American Society of Anesthesiologists, Park Ridge, Illinois.

V. Patient Monitoring

During N_2O/O_2 sedation it is necessary to continuously monitor the patient. This is to ensure a positive experience for the patient and to discover adverse reactions quickly. The ASA Task Force recommends that monitoring the patient include evaluating level of consciousness, pulmonary ventilation, oxygenation, and hemodynamics.

A. Level of consciousness can be monitored by the patient's response to verbal stimulation. Monitoring level of consciousness reduces risks associated with moderate sedation.

B. Monitoring ventilatory function can be accomplished by observation or auscultation. This reduces the risk of adverse outcomes associated with moderate sedation. A great advantage of N_2O/O_2 delivery is the reservoir bag. This serves as a supplemental supply of O_2 for the patient but also is a valid method of monitoring a patient's respiration. The bag mimics respiratory excursions, allowing the practitioner to monitor the frequency and depth of respirations with a reliable visual source.

C. Pulse oximetry detects oxygen desaturation and can uncover early hypoxemia. Early detection of hypoxemia through the use of a pulse oximeter decreases the likelihood of severe adverse reactions. Cyanosis is a late sign of respiratory distress.

D. Intraoperative monitoring of vital signs is highly recommended during moderate sedation.[1,9] Regular monitoring of vital signs reduces the likelihood of adverse outcomes. During moderate sedation, vital signs should be measured every 5 minutes.

VI. Emergency Preparedness

A. Personnel preparation
1. Persons who are involved in the administration and monitoring of minimal and/or moderate sedation using N_2O should understand the pharmacokinetics of the drug and be able to recognize complications.
2. Personnel who use N_2O/O_2 sedation should also be certified in basic life support that includes CPR and management of airway obstruction for adults, children, and infants.[9]
B. Emergency equipment
1. Appropriate emergency equipment should be readily available wherever N_2O is administered. The ASA Task Force recommends that an automated external defibrillator should be available when moderate sedation is intended.[1]
2. Additional equipment that is recommended includes antagonist medications, a positive-pressure ventilation system, adequate suction to clear an airway, advanced airway equipment, and resuscitation medications.[1,9]
3. These items are standard for those who administer sedation.

REFERENCES

1. ASA Task Force: Practice guidelines for sedation and analgesia by non-anesthesiologists, *Anesthesiology* 96(4):1004, 2002.
2. Wolfe S: The practical approach to painless dentistry, *Dentistry Today* 11:30, 1992.
3. American Society of Anesthesiologists: New classification of physical status, *Anesthesiology* 24:111, 1963.
4. Sweitzer B: *Handbook of preoperative assessment and treatment*, Philadelphia, 2000, Lippincott Williams & Wilkins.
5. American Academy of Pediatric Dentistry: Standards for basic intraoperative monitoring, *ASA Newsletter* 50:13, 1986.
6. American Association of Oral and Maxillofacial Surgeons, Committee on Anesthesia: *Office anesthesia evaluation manual*, ed 4, Rosemont, Ill, 1991, The Association.
7. American Academy of Pediatric Dentistry: Guidelines for the elective use of conscious sedation, deep sedation, and general anesthesia in pediatric patients, *Pediatrics* 76:317, 1985.
8. American Academy of Periodontology: Subcommittee on Anxiety and Pain Control of the Pharmacotherapeutics Committee: *Guidelines for the use of conscious sedation in periodontics*, Chicago, 1990, The Association.
9. American Dental Association, Council on Dental Education and Licensure: *Guidelines for the use of conscious sedation, deep sedation, and general anesthesia for dentists*, Chicago, 2002, American Dental Association.
10. Theil D: Personal communication, October 2002.
11. Malamed SF: Sedation: a guide to patient management, ed 4, St Louis, 2003, Mosby, p 65.

11
Titration of N_2O/O_2 Gases

Titration is a method of administering a drug in incremental amounts until a desired endpoint is reached (Box 11-1). For N_2O/O_2 sedation, N_2O is given in incremental doses until a patient has reached a comfortable, relaxed state of sedation. The ability to titrate N_2O is a significant advantage because it allows the specific amount of drug that is required by that patient to be delivered. If titration is done properly, the patient does not receive any more of the drug than is necessary. Occasionally patients have had negative experiences with N_2O/O_2 sedation. In such cases, the operator most likely did not titrate the amount of N_2O necessary to make the patient comfortable; instead, the patient received an inappropriately large amount of drug, which usually causes oversedation. The concept of titration is the single most important skill to be learned by the operator to be a competent, safe administrator of any drug by any route, including N_2O (Figure 11-1). *The titration technique is regarded as the current standard of care when administering N_2O/O_2 for sedation.*

Using a "fixed dose" or the so-called rapid induction technique for N_2O/O_2 administration has been advocated by some clinicians for years. This technique involves administering a large quantity of N_2O (up to 50%) initially to patients, particularly children. Although advocates of this technique maintain it is necessary to quickly calm an intensely fearful or uncooperative child, this technique can also result in increased fear and continued disruptive behavior that may be accompanied by nausea and vomiting. In addition, because clinicians often do not allow the parent or guardian to accompany the child in the operatory, it is likely that parents will be unaware that their child has had a negative experience. Pinkham[1] describes so well in the text *Pediatric Dentistry: Infancy through Adolescence,* that using high concentrations with a rapid administration technique produces many negative effects. The use of a 50% N_2O and 50% O_2 product has also become a common practice for some. Seasoned clinicians and researchers Gillman and Lichtigfeld[2] advocate the use of the titration technique and advise others that they may have improved success rates when using this technique instead of a 50% premixed concentration. It is therefore recommended that the rapid induction of high concentrations of N_2O not be used with adults and only with children under specific conditions and by a trained pediatric clinician.

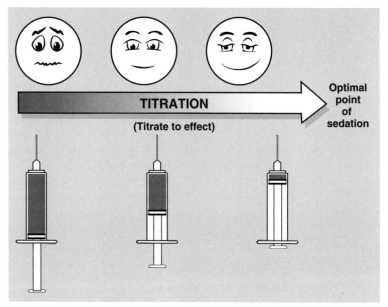

Figure 11-1   Titration is the incremental dosing of a drug. Incremental doses of a drug are administered to achieve an optimal point of sedation.

BOX 11-1
Titration Is...

a method of drug administration in which definitive amounts of the substance are given in incremental doses until a specific endpoint is reached.

I. Significance

A. Provide proper amount of a drug. It is extremely desirable to provide only the amount of a drug necessary for the procedure being performed. This allows for the expeditious elimination of the drug from the system, but more importantly, it creates a positive experience for the patient. With careful titration, vigilant monitoring of the patient, and updated equipment, negative experiences with N_2O/O_2 sedation should be rare.

B. Titration is very important when administering any drug. It minimizes the chances of a severe, possibly life-threatening reaction should the patient be allergic to the drug. Fortunately, since the discovery of N_2O, no allergic reaction to the drug has been reported.

C. Titration allows for biologic variability. It is essential to treat each patient as an individual, taking into account the concept of individual biovariability.

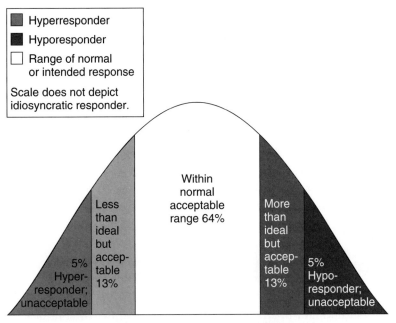

Figure 11-2   Range of individual biovariability.

This concept is based on the premise that no two individuals react the same way in response to a drug or treatment modality. What works for one will not necessarily work for another, nor will one patient respond in the same way on different days.

1. As each drug is initially tested, researchers commonly find a small percentage of hyporesponders and hyperresponders. Certain people will have no effect from an optimal dose of the drug, whereas some will incur dramatic effects. A drug is useful when the desired outcome occurs in a large majority of the population without unwanted side effects. Figure 11-2 depicts the range of individual biovariability.

2. Individual biovariability holds true for nonpharmacologic methods as well. It is wise to keep an open, informed mind when experimenting with pain and anxiety management options.

3. No two humans are alike, and the same individual may give a different response on any given day. For example, habitually dispensing 10 mg diazepam (Valium), 50 mg meperidine (Demerol), or using 40% N$_2$O as a "usual" dose must be avoided because patient response cannot be guaranteed.

D. Sometimes idiosyncratic (unpredictable) reactions may be encountered that are untoward and inexplicable (e.g., excitement after receiving a sedative drug). Titrating the drug uncovers such responses and minimizes unexpected reactions immediately (Box 11-2).

E. Application to other drugs. Titration can be applied to other drugs as well. For example, staggering local anesthetic injections over time allows for bio-

---

BOX 11-2
Advantages of N₂O Titration

- Only the amount of drug required by the patient is given
- Allows for individual biovariability
- Uncovers idiosyncratic reactions early
- Minimizes negative experiences with oversedation

---

transformation tailored to the procedure and the patient's physiology. Titrating the dose of a drug is the considerate way to treat a patient individually. Titrating a drug to the appropriate level of sedation is a valuable learned skill.

II. Adjusting Levels Appropriately

A. A great advantage of N_2O is the ability to adjust levels of sedation. Because of this important pharmacologic property, the onset of clinical effects is rapid. Signs and symptoms of sedation may be missed if close attention is not given.

B. Titration also allows for prolonged procedures to be accomplished effectively.
   1. For example, when a potentially painful phase of treatment approaches, the N_2O gas may be increased. And conversely, as the intensity of the treatment subsides the N_2O gas can be decreased.
   2. As the procedure nears completion, amounts of N_2O being delivered should be minimal. Because a minimum of 5 minutes of postoxygenation is required, it is appropriate to terminate the flow of N_2O and deliver 100% O_2 before completion of the procedure.

C. Remember that because of individual biovariability patients will require different levels of N_2O on different days and for different procedures.
   1. The percentage of N_2O noted in a patient's chart from the last visit is not relevant for the current appointment.
   2. The most common mistake made with N_2O/O_2 sedation is to automatically deliver a preset percentage of N_2O to a patient.
   3. Negative patient experiences from N_2O/O_2 sedation are most likely because the patient was oversedated as a result of operator error. Far too often patients blame any negative experience on the drug itself.

REFERENCES
1. Pinkham JR, Casamassimo PS, McTigue DJ, Fields HW, Nowak A: *Pediatric dentistry: infancy through adolescence*, ed 3, Philadelphia, 1999, WB Saunders.
2. Gillman MA, Lichtigfeld FJ: Analgesic nitrous oxide: an opioid treatment for migraine, *Am J Emer Med* 18(4):501, 2000.

12

Signs and Symptoms of N_2O/O_2 Sedation

Individual biovariability accounts for different reactions to various amounts of N_2O. Some individuals experience several symptoms; others only a few. Symptoms are intense for some and insignificant for others. There are instances when signs are obvious; other times signs are subtle. It is extremely important that the clinician knows what signs and symptoms to look for when administering and monitoring N_2O/O_2 sedation. Keeping a constant vigil is imperative because pleasant sensations may quickly become unpleasant. Knowledge of the appropriate technique and associated physical, physiologic, and psychologic changes increases the practitioner's confidence with this procedure and minimizes negative patient experiences. The ultimate goal is to increase patient comfort through relaxation.

I. Appropriate Minimal Sedation

A. A desirable level of sedation for both patient and operator (minimal sedation) can be achieved by using the titration-time technique plus careful monitoring of the patient's signs and symptoms. Certain physical, physiologic, and psychologic effects may manifest in individuals when N_2O and O_2 are administered (Box 12-1).

B. It is imperative that the operator recognizes when the desired effects are reached, for it is then that an appropriate level of sedation is accomplished and administration of additional drug is not necessary. The operator must watch closely for the following:

1. Psychologic signs
   a. The patient is relaxed and comfortable (Figure 12-1).
   b. If asked, the patient acknowledges a reduced sense of fear and anxiety.
   c. The patient's mood may be categorized as happy, pleasant, satisfied, or even ambivalent (Figure 12-2).
2. Body movement
   a. Relaxation may be expressed overtly or inadvertently through physical movements.
   b. Patients usually take deeper respirations when they are relaxed.
3. Eyes
   a. The activity of the patient's eyes is a good indicator of the level of sedation. With experience, the operator will often be able to make

Figure 12-1   The patient is relaxed and comfortable.

accurate judgments about the level of sedation by looking at the patient's eyes.
  b. Initially, during preparatory steps, patients' eyes will be active. Patients will be alert and their eyes will follow the operator's actions and movements.
  c. As sedation commences, the activity of the patient's eyes will begin to slow. Eye movement will be reduced and blink rate will be slower (Figure 12-3).
  d. As sedation continues, there will be a point, often, when the eyes may appear "glazed" or "glassy."
 4. Facial expression
  a. Patients who are appropriately sedated are content.
  b. There should not be signs of tension on the patient's face.

BOX 12-1

Signs and Symptoms of Appropriate Minimal Sedation

Patient is comfortable and relaxed
Patient acknowledges reduced fear and anxiety
Patient is aware of surroundings
Patient responds to directions and conversation
Protective cough and gag reflexes remain intact
Eyes become less active and glazed look appears
Patient may experience:
    Tingling in extremities and/or near mouth
    Heaviness in legs and arms
    Body warmth
    Light feeling
    Vasodilation in face and neck

Figure 12-2   The patient is in a positive mood.

Figure 12-3   The patient's eye movement will be reduced.

5. Awareness
   a. When appropriately sedated, patients are fully conscious and aware of their surroundings. With relaxation, patients' surroundings are no longer threatening and patients will have a sense of well-being.
   b. Patients will be able to respond rationally and coherently to the operator's inquiry or directions. They can maintain conversation. With

minimal sedation, protective cough and gag reflexes remain intact. It is important to stress that patients refrain from talking in order to receive the drug's effects and minimize contamination of the environment.

   c. If a local anesthetic injection is given during the procedure, the operator can test the patient's level of sedation by asking, "Would this be a good time to give you the injection?" Patients will affirm the injection can be given when they are appropriately sedated and will be accepting of the procedure. Anecdotally, the success of this questioning has proven to be quite reliable in clinical practice.

6. Other physiologic signs and symptoms

   a. Patients should not be given specific physical signs to expect such as tingling in the fingers, toes, cheeks, lips, tongue, head, or chest area. Some patients experience tingling sensations but others may not. Therefore the operator should not pose questions as to the presence of this symptom. Patients may think they are not being affected by the drug because they lack this symptom. Questions should be goal-oriented, focusing on *how* the patient is feeling rather than *what* the patient is feeling.

   b. There may be noted heaviness in the patient's thighs and/or legs. Conversely, some patients experience a lighter feeling in their extremities.

   c. Because of the drug's effect on the tympanic membrane, the patient's voice may resonate or carry a hypernasal tone. In addition, the patient may sense that the operator's voice is farther away and therefore harder to hear. Fabijan et al[1] challenge the idea that hearing acuity is changed with low levels of N_2O but they indicate that the perception of the loudness of sounds is diminished.

   d. Patients may notice they feel warm. Their cheeks and/or neck may flush as vasodilation occurs.

II. Oversedation

A. Discomfort in patients. As N_2O concentrations are increased, the signs and symptoms of comfort and relaxation may disappear. Some sensations may continue to be tolerable but become intense. Sometimes, changes in patient comfort occur rapidly and a patient can suddenly become very uncomfortable. In either case, the patient is no longer in a relaxed state. When a patient becomes uncomfortable in any way, it is important to decrease N_2O concentrations immediately. It is critical to regain patient comfort as soon as possible to avoid a significant negative experience.

B. Signs and symptoms. Signs and symptoms of oversedation may not always be visually obvious. The operator should always be present whenever N_2O is being delivered to continuously monitor the patient. Patients should be told to signal or tell the operator if, at any point, they become uncomfortable. In addition, the operator should be asking questions of patients periodically to

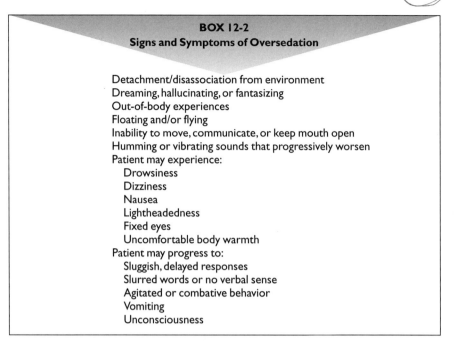

BOX 12-2
Signs and Symptoms of Oversedation

Detachment/disassociation from environment
Dreaming, hallucinating, or fantasizing
Out-of-body experiences
Floating and/or flying
Inability to move, communicate, or keep mouth open
Humming or vibrating sounds that progressively worsen
Patient may experience:
    Drowsiness
    Dizziness
    Nausea
    Lightheadedness
    Fixed eyes
    Uncomfortable body warmth
Patient may progress to:
    Sluggish, delayed responses
    Slurred words or no verbal sense
    Agitated or combative behavior
    Vomiting
    Unconsciousness

Figure 12-4   Oversedation; patient is irritated and uncomfortable.

assess comfort. The following are examples of the signs and symptoms of oversedation (Box 12-2).
1. Psychologic signs
    a. The relaxed, comfortable state has disappeared.
        i. Patients may indicate that they just don't feel the same and that the effects such as tingling have intensified. This feeling may be annoying but not uncomfortable (Figure 12-4).

      ii. Or, the patient may indicate a sudden, very uncomfortable feeling in which symptoms are intolerable.

  b. In some cases, the patient may actually begin dreaming and/or hallucinating. Patients may attempt to respond to voices, people, visual effects, etc.

  c. Sexual fantasizing may occur with oversedation. The ramifications of this occurrence are discussed in Chapter 18.

2. Body movement
   a. Patients may show signs of being agitated or physically uncomfortable. They may become restless and fidgety.
   b. Patients can possibly become combative and/or violent.
   c. Patients can also become very sluggish with their motions or unable to move their extremities.

3. Eyes
   a. The eyes of an oversedated patient can become fixed and nonresponsive.
   b. Heavily sedated patients often want to sleep and have difficulty keeping their eyes open.
   c. Occasionally, patients indicate their field of vision narrows. The area of their peripheral vision becomes black. Patients may comment that they feel like they are "blacking out."

4. Facial expression
   a. Fits of uncontrolled laughter are a sign of oversedation. When this occurs, the patient primarily mouth-breathes, which changes the level of sedation.
   b. After the patient becomes calm and nose breathing resumes, a roller coaster sedation effect may occur and nausea can ensue.

5. Awareness
   a. Patients may no longer feel that they are in the same surroundings. A detachment or disassociation from the environment is possible.
   b. Often patients indicate lightweight, floating or flying sensations. These may accompany the environmental detachment.
   c. Disassociation or out-of-body experiences can occur.

6. Other physiologic signs and symptoms
   a. Patients' perception of their hearing may change. The patient may perceive normal sounds as very intense. Humming noises or vibrations in their ears may simply be distracting or become bothersome.
   b. The pleasant warmth felt in earlier states may intensify and become uncomfortable. The patient may express various signs of being too warm or even hot. Wanting to loosen a collar or roll up sleeves may be indicators of perceived temperature increase.
   c. The patient may become very drowsy, which is not to be confused with being relaxed. The patient may actually want to sleep or appear to be in a dreamlike state.
   d. Words may be slurred or repeated; sentences may not be coherent. The patient may not be able to respond to verbal commands.
   e. Dizziness, lightheadedness, and spinning sensations are common in oversedation. This may produce transient nausea for some people.

C. Oversedation can produce physical and physiologic effects that are serious, if not life threatening.
   1. Vomiting may occur with oversedation.
      a. Vomiting occurs more readily in children.
      b. Silent regurgitation is a type of action in which vomitus reaches the level of the epiglottis and can lead to aspiration into the lungs. This situation demands immediate advanced medical attention.
   2. The patient can actually become unconscious. Although this is difficult to do because of the pharmacokinetics of N_2O, all healthcare personnel must be able to respond to this type of emergency (see Chapter 8).
   3. *These situations can easily be prevented using the titration technique with continuous monitoring.*
D. When a patient has a pleasant experience using N_2O/O_2 sedation and the goal of analgesia and reduced anxiety is reached, success is achieved. However, oversedation typically produces a negative experience. Oversedation is likely when an inappropriate technique (i.e., fixed-dose, rapid induction) is applied or when equipment is used that only delivers a preset amount of drug. Patients who have had negative experiences with N_2O will, most often, not want to use the drug again. Conscientious, educated practitioners will not allow oversedation to destroy the capability of this drug to remain a viable option for pain and anxiety management.

REFERENCE

1. Fabijan DJ et al: The effect of nitrous oxide on hearing, *Anaesth Intensive Care* 28(3):270, 2000.

13

Technique for N₂O/O₂ Administration

The basic principles of N_2O/O_2 administration have been developed from decades of experience. Adhering to these principles helps to ensure a positive experience for both the patient and the operator. Titrating the drug and careful observation of patient response are keys to successful administration. It is extremely important to know the fundamentals of the technique for administering N_2O/O_2. If these basic principles are followed, it is likely that the experience will be positive for both the operator and the patient. In the past these basic principles have not been followed, and too frequently negative patient experiences resulted. Concomitantly, operator frustration and lack of confidence occurred. It may take several positive experiences for a patient to become convinced that previous uncomfortable experiences were caused not by the N_2O but rather by its method of administration. The technique is not difficult; titrating the drug while observing patient response is the key to success.

I. Fundamental Principles for Appropriate Administration

A. The operator should be enthusiastic and confident that the experience will be positive. This attitude will transfer to the patient.

B. Confidence is primarily preparation reflected in the individual who is informed and educated about N_2O pharmacokinetics. Be knowledgeable about what N_2O can and cannot accomplish.

C. Recognize that a patient in your care represents the best opportunity you have to express genuine care and concern. Patients are more likely to refer others to you after a good experience.

D. Informed consent must be obtained from each patient before each N_2O/O_2 administration.

E. The amount of N_2O required by a patient on any given day or time varies. Do not adopt the fixed-dose philosophy; the amount of N_2O required on the previous visit is not relevant for this appointment (see Chapter 11).

F. The procedure begins and ends with 100% pure O_2.

G. The patient should not be left alone. The effects of CNS depression may be quick and/or subtle; constant monitoring must be done by a professional trained in N_2O/O_2 sedation. Remember, you are responsible for the effects that occur at the intended level of sedation and the next (deeper) level. Refer to the ASA Practice Guidelines for Sedation and Analgesia by Non-Anesthesiologists.

H. Accurate documentation of all procedures, reactions, complications, etc. must be maintained in the patient's file.

I. Because the final objective of the procedure is patient comfort, the patient should be placed in a comfortable position.
   1. To begin, depending on the discipline and the area of the body to be treated, the patient should be relaxed in a basic physiologic position.
   2. The upper torso should be slightly reclined and the legs slightly elevated. This can be easily accomplished with an adjustable chair. If a bed is used, prop the patient's head with pillows.

J. Maintain open communication with the patient. Sedated patients may not be able to accurately state their feelings. Specific questions are necessary to assess the patient. For example, you may ask, "Are you uncomfortable?" or "On a scale of 1 to 10, what is your level of discomfort?"

K. If N_2O/O_2 is to be given at a subsequent appointment, advise the patient to avoid eating a big meal before that appointment. The presence of stomach contents does not precipitate vomiting; however, if vomiting occurs, there is risk for aspiration. The propensity for vomiting is higher in children than in adults.[1] Refer to Chapter 10 for specific ASA recommended fasting guidelines.

II. Preoperative Unit Preparation

A. The N_2O/O_2 sedation armamentarium should include all equipment necessary to provide safe sedation experiences for the patient and a safe environment for the operator and all other exposed personnel.
   1. This equipment should be current, accurate, and include all available components for minimizing trace gas contamination.
   2. Equipment will include an accurate flowmeter, scavenging masks, and a vacuum system able to eliminate gases at a rate of at least 45 L per minute.[2]

B. Ensure vacuum and ventilation exhaust are vented to the outside; make sure they are not near fresh-air intake vents.[2]

C. Assess the room and area ventilation.[2] The recirculation of room air, such as air conditioning, is not recommended. A ventilation system with a fresh air exchange system ensures that waste gases are not circulated elsewhere within the building. Fresh air exchanges can also be provided by opening a window or door. Use oscillating room fans near the floor to sweep waste gases out of the area and/or to the outside.

D. Confirm the absence of leaks at pressure connections on the unit. Bubbles will appear at leaking locations when a soap and water solution is used.
   1. This procedure is recommended each time a cylinder is changed.
   2. High-pressure lines should also be assessed periodically. The ADA expert panel recommends that this be done quarterly.[2]
   3. Inspect the conducting tubing, reservoir bag, and their connections for leaks. These rubber products are subject to UV light degradation and should be visually inspected before each use. New silicone products appear to be more durable.

E. Connect proper parts to unit.
   1. Connect conducting tubing and reservoir bag to the unit if they are not already in place.
   2. A bag barrier may be used to cover the unit; however, make sure the flowmeter can be easily read and knobs are easily accessible through the barrier.
F. Open both the O_2 and N_2O cylinders.
   1. Turn the knob counterclockwise on the top of the large cylinders used in a central gas supply system. Open the stem valves on the top of smaller cylinders associated with portable systems using the wrench provided with the equipment (Figure 13-1).
   2. The pressure-gauge indicators (Figure 13-2) will rise and stop. Again, the O_2 gauge will give an accurate indication of the amount of gas in the tank. The N_2O pressure gauge will read approximately 750 psi unless the tank is nearly empty (Figure 13-3).
   3. If there is no O_2, the machine is nonfunctional. O_2 must be available at all times for the N_2O to flow.
   4. A central supply manifold will automatically switch the system to a full O_2 tank should one become depleted (Figure 13-4). If no additional O_2 is available for a central system, an alarm will sound or indicator light will flash on the system monitor. If there is no gas for the system, the lack of O_2 will automatically stop the flow of N_2O and gas will cease flowing to the patient. Lights will stop flashing or floating balls will drop on the flowmeter.
   5. The operator managing a portable system has to visually monitor the O_2 pressure gauge and manually replace cylinders when the oxygen supply is

Figure 13-1   Open the O_2 tank by turning the valve on top of the cylinder.

Figure 13-2   O₂ pressure gauge indicating cylinder contents.

Figure 13-3   N₂O pressure gauge indicating cylinder contents.

getting low. It is important to have a second cylinder readily available and opened before the oxygen is completely depleted to prevent loss of patient sedation.

G. Make sure the master switch on the flowmeter is in the "on" position.

H. Activate the main portion of the scavenging system by turning on the suction or evacuation system to the appropriate level.

Figure 13-4   Pressure gauges on manifold. (Courtesy Porter Instrument Co.)

1. This level may be automatically preset for some central supply systems. In this case no further adjustments are necessary.
2. In some central supply systems it is necessary to attach the end of the conduction tubing into the suction at the operatory.
3. For portable systems, it is necessary to place the tubing end into the high-speed suction (Figure 13–5).
4. If manual adjustment of the suction is necessary, create enough flow to prevent waste gas from entering the atmosphere. Manufacturing companies are currently marketing monitoring devices that indicate the optimal evacuation level of 45 L per minute. Devices may be mounted close to the flowmeter; others may be found at the end of the conduction tubing before it is placed into the vacuum. Floating balls or dials on these devices indicate the appropriate amount of suction (Figure 13-6).
I. Push the O_2 flush button until the reservoir bag is partially inflated to approximately two-thirds full (Figure 13-7, *A*). Inflation of the bag is evaluated again when establishing appropriate flow to the patient (Figure 13-7, *B*).

Figure 13-5   Engaging the delivery unit to the evacuation system.

Figure 13-6   **A** and **B,** Adjust suction level according to manufacturer's system. (**A,** Courtesy Accutron, Inc.; **B,** Courtesy, Porter Instrument Company.)

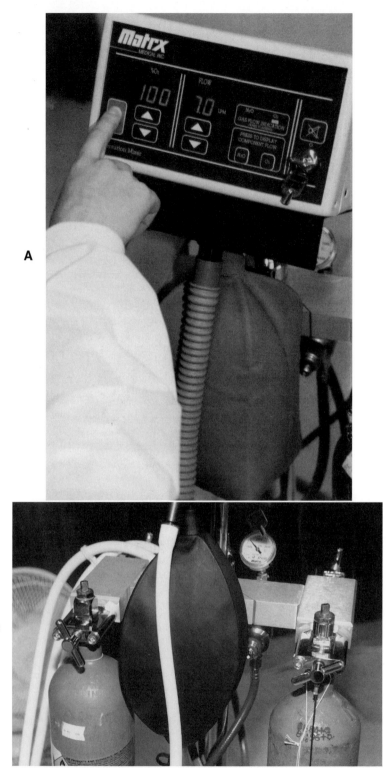

Figure 13-7   **A** and **B,** Fill the reservoir bag two-thirds full using the O$_2$ flush button.

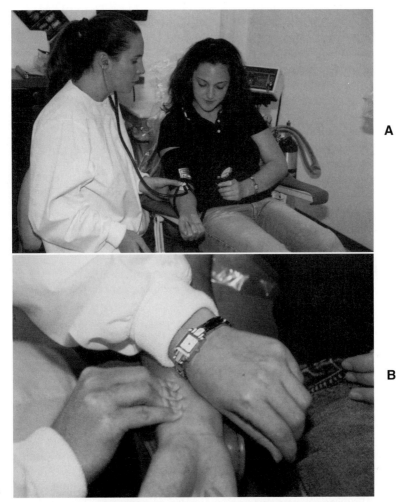

Figure 13-8   A and **B,** Obtain blood pressure reading and pulse rate.

III. Patient Participation

A. Measure the baseline vital signs of blood pressure (Figure 13-8, *A*), pulse (Figure 13-8, *B*), and respirations. Record these values on the sedation record or in the patient's chart.

B. Select the appropriate size and type of scavenging breathing apparatus for the patient. If using a nasal hood, find the size and/or scent most desirable to the patient. If using a full face mask, select the appropriate size. Attach breathing apparatus to conduction tubing.

C. Begin O$_2$ flow to the nasal hood or mask. The ball will float or the light will appear on the O$_2$ side of the flowmeter.

D. Estimate the total liters flow per minute (L/min) according to the size and physical and physiologic condition of the patient.

Figure 13-9 Establish the appropriate tidal volume for the patient.

1. For an average-size adult, begin with 6 to 7 L/min (Figure 13-9). It is best to err with more flow than needed initially to avoid a suffocating feeling. As the patient becomes relaxed, you may find that less flow is adequate.
2. Begin with 4 to 5 L/min for most children.
3. Set the machine to deliver 100% O_2 at the level of liters per minute that you have initially chosen. To ensure that there is flow, listen for the sound of O_2 moving into the breathing apparatus.

E. Place nasal hood or face mask on patient. Ask the patient to assist you in obtaining a snug but comfortable fit.
   1. Instruct the patient to adjust it at any time throughout the procedure. Allowing patients this option gives them a sense of control.
   2. Adjust the conducting tubes behind the patient's head to ensure a snug fit (Figure 13-10). This will decrease the amount of air leaking from the mask.
      a. Take care not to tighten the apparatus so that patient movement is prohibited or pressure marks appear on the face.
      b. A piece of gauze may be folded over the patient's nose to minimize gas leakage should adjustment be inadequate.
   3. Not only does an improper fit waste gas, but trace gas leakage contaminates the clinician's immediate environment (breathing zone).

F. Determine the appropriate tidal volume needed for the patient using the flow of 100% O_2.
   1. Ask patients if the flow is sufficient to enable them to breathe comfortably. Also determine if the patient feels that there is gas leaking out of the mask.
   2. The reservoir bag is a good indicator for appropriate flow[2] (Box 13-1).

Figure 13-10   Secure the nasal hood to the patient.

Figure 13-11   Reduce the tidal volume if the reservoir bag is bulging.

a. If the bag is bulging (Figure 13-11), the patient, most likely, is not breathing as much gas as is flowing from the machine. The extra gas is being retained in the bag causing it to overinflate. It is also possible that the patient is mouth-breathing. Often, breathing pattern becomes more normal and relaxed once the patient becomes familiar with the nasal hood.

b. Turn down the O_2 level (L/min) until the bag deflates to about two-thirds full.

Figure 13-12   Be aware of potential problems, such as kinking hoses.

| **BOX 13-1** |
| **Determining Appropriate Gas Flow in Liters per Minute (L/min) Before Titrating N₂O** |

Begin at an average flow of 6 to 8 L/min O_2 for an adult or 4 to 6 L/min for a child.
If the reservoir bag flattens, fill it again using the O_2 flush valve and increase the flow by 1 to 2 L/min.
If the reservoir bag balloons, decrease the flow by 1 to 2 L/min.

c. If the bag continues to inflate like a balloon, it is possible that flow has been blocked somehow (Figure 13-12). Sometimes the bag may get caught between cylinders or the nonrebreathing valve may stick. Attend to this situation quickly.

d. If the bag is collapsing, then the patient is breathing all of the flow coming from the machine plus the reserve stored in the reservoir bag. In this case, increase the liters flow per minute to the patient. It will be necessary to reinflate the reservoir bag using the O_2 flush button (Figure 13-13).

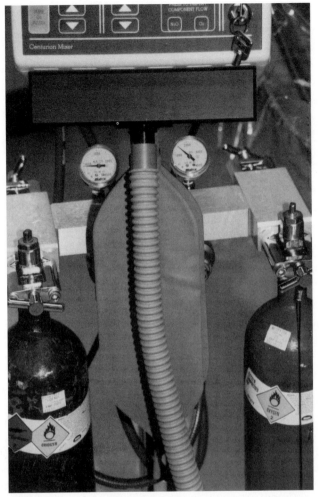

Figure 13-13   Increase the tidal volume if the reservoir bag collapses.

G. Constant flow per minute. Once appropriate total liters flow per minute has been established, this amount will remain constant for the duration of the procedure.

IV. Administration of N_2O

A. Administration technique. Depending on the type of machine, there may be slight variations in the administration technique.
  1. If there are two controls on the machine that independently adjust the levels of each gas, the operator will have to *manually* adjust both the O_2 and the N_2O during administration. Each time N_2O is added, the

Figure 13-14   Sedation machine with independent N₂O and O₂ controls.

amount of O_2 will have to be decreased to keep the total liters flow per minute constant (Figure 13-14).

2. Some machines *automatically* decrease the amount of O_2 whenever N_2O is added to keep the established flow constant (Figure 13-15).

3. No matter what type of machine is being used, it is important to keep the established liters flow per minute constant throughout the procedure.

a. On machines that are digital, the LED number displayed indicates the total liters flow per minute.

b. On machines with dual tubes and floating balls, total liters flow is calculated by adding the numbers from both sides of the flowmeter at the level of the middle of a floating ball. For example, 2 L/min N_2O + 5 L/min O_2 = 7 total liters flow per minute (Figure 13-16).

c. The number associated with a floating ball does not indicate the percentage of N_2O being delivered. For example, 2 L/min N_2O *does not equal* 20% N_2O.

d. The actual percentage of N_2O is calculated by dividing the N_2O L/min by the total L/min. For example,

$$\frac{2\ L/min\ N_2O}{7\ L/min} = 28.5\%\ N_2O$$

e. N_2O percentages have been calculated for you and are available for your convenience in Appendix B. They may be photocopied, laminated, and attached to your machine, or placed in your operatory.

f. On machines that have the percent of O_2 displayed, it is necessary to subtract the number from 100% to obtain the percent of N_2O being delivered. For example, when 60% O_2 is displayed, 40% N_2O is being delivered.

Figure 13-15   Sedation machine that keeps tidal volume constant and adjusts gases according to percent administered.

B. *The administration technique of titrating N_2O is recognized as the standard of care* (Box 13-2). Slow titration of small doses of drug is critical to prevent oversedation (Figure 13-17).

C. There is not an exact amount of N_2O that is required to be delivered during the titration technique.

　1. However, a recommended regimen is to begin with approximately 10% N_2O or 1 L, and add N_2O thereafter in increments of 5% or 0.5 L with a 60-second (1-minute) minimum between increments (Box 13-3).

　2. When beginning to add N_2O, it is preferable to wait at least 60 seconds (1 minute) after a dose before adding the next increment.

　3. When sedation is becoming evident, it is recommended to wait longer (up to 3 minutes) between doses to prevent oversedation. This can occur

Figure 13-16 Tidal volume displayed does not indicate percentage of N₂O delivered. (Courtesy Porter Instrument Co.)

Figure 13-17 N₂O/O₂ Administration = Titration + Time.

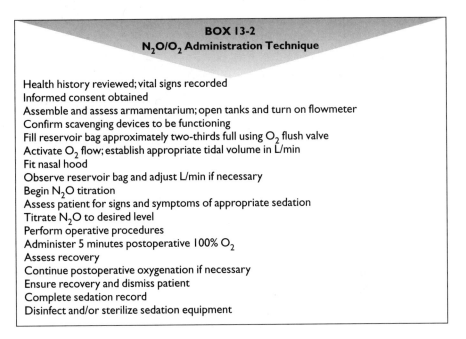

BOX 13-2
N_2O/O_2 Administration Technique

Health history reviewed; vital signs recorded
Informed consent obtained
Assemble and assess armamentarium; open tanks and turn on flowmeter
Confirm scavenging devices to be functioning
Fill reservoir bag approximately two-thirds full using O_2 flush valve
Activate O_2 flow; establish appropriate tidal volume in L/min
Fit nasal hood
Observe reservoir bag and adjust L/min if necessary
Begin N_2O titration
Assess patient for signs and symptoms of appropriate sedation
Titrate N_2O to desired level
Perform operative procedures
Administer 5 minutes postoperative 100% O_2
Assess recovery
Continue postoperative oxygenation if necessary
Ensure recovery and dismiss patient
Complete sedation record
Disinfect and/or sterilize sedation equipment

BOX 13-3
N_2O/O_2 Administration Technique Using Titration

Begin with approximately 10% or about 1 L of N_2O.
Increase in increments of 5% or approximately 0.5 L every 1 to 3 minutes until sedation becomes apparent.
Wait longer between increments when desired level of sedation is near. This prevents oversedation and maximizes patient comfort.

easily when doses are administered too close together with insufficient time for peak effect of one dose to take place before another dose is given.

4. Instruct the patient to breathe through the nose when using a nasal hood and to keep the lips sealed (Figure 13-18). This allows for a more accurate level of sedation and gives the clinician a better idea of when an appropriate level is reached. If the patient is talking excessively or verbalizing answers to clinician questioning during administration of N_2O doses, it is likely that oversedation could occur when the patient resumes nasal breathing. Also, mouth breathing and/or talking are a major source of ambient air contamination.

D. Watch patient comfort level. Titrate to a level of sedation that is determined by patient comfort and relaxation. Watch closely for the signs and symptoms of ideal sedation.

Figure 13-18   When administering N$_2$O/O$_2$, have patient breathe through the nose.

1. Remember, there is no preset percentage for N$_2$O/O$_2$ sedation for a given patient or experience. A fixed-dose technique does not represent the current standard of care.
2. The percentage of N$_2$O administered to a patient for a given experience will, most likely, not be the same for any subsequent experience. Individual biovariability accounts for this variation in amount. Using a prescribed or previously administered amount may oversedate the patient and cause a negative experience unfairly blamed on the N$_2$O.
E. Intraoperative monitoring includes vigilant observation of the patient's responses and reactions in addition to observation of the reservoir bag.
  1. The reservoir bag serves as a monitor of the patient's respirations. The bag inflates and deflates slightly with the patient's inhalations and exhalations. Use this as a sign of depth, rate, and reflection of lung activity.
  2. Cumulative effects of N$_2$O may be seen as the duration of delivery increases. The level of sedation may deepen, resulting in uncomfortable symptoms for the patient. Ask patients periodically how they are feeling.
  3. Levels of sedation may be influenced if the patient is allowed to maintain conversation and breathe through the mouth. Therefore, patient talking should be kept to a minimum.
F. Perform necessary procedures (Figure 13-19). The goal is to keep the patient relaxed and comfortable.
  1. Adjust the level of N$_2$O as needed depending on the intensity of the procedures and the responses of the patient.
  2. You may decrease the N$_2$O incrementally to a lesser amount for certain nonstimulating phases of treatment or completely if you are nearing completion of treatment.
G. When you terminate the N$_2$O flow, continue delivering 100% O$_2$ during final minutes of the operative procedure. This begins your required postoperative oxygenation period of 5 minutes minimum. It is vital to pay close attention to this minimum time (Figure 13-20).

1. It is unnecessary and inappropriate to use the O_2 flush button to remove the admixture of gases from the bag to provide 100% O_2, because this contaminates the environment with N_2O. The technique of lifting the nasal hood off of the patient and purging the contents of the reservoir bag by squeezing it (Figure 13-21) represents an inappropriate technique and is not recommended.[2]
2. To begin the postoperative oxygenation period of 100% O_2, simply terminate the flow of N_2O and continue the flow of O_2.

Figure 13-19   Perform procedures when patient is appropriately sedated.

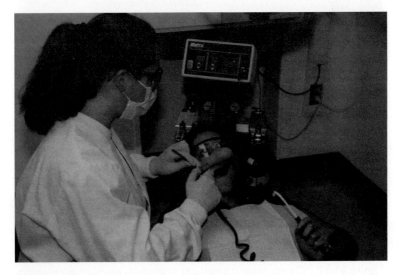

Figure 13-20   Begin postoperative oxygenation (5-minute minimum) near the completion of procedure.

3. If you administer O_2 for the required time during the final nonintensive phase of the procedure, the patient may be assessed as soon as the procedure is completed and dismissed rather than having to wait for the postoperative oxygenation period to begin.

H. Assess the recovery of the patient. See Chapter 14 for specific details on recovery procedures.

1. If the patient senses any lethargy, dizziness, lightheadedness, or headache, continue 100% O_2 for additional minutes. Continue 100% O_2 for as long as is necessary (Figure 13-22).

2. When, and only when, the patient feels normal, you can remove the breathing apparatus and allow the patient to breathe room air.

I. Obtain postoperative vital sign measurements. Extend your appreciation of the patient's cooperation and trust. Reinforce the success of the appointment, then dismiss the patient (Figures 13-23 and 13-24).

J. A condensed version of the administration technique can be found in Appendix E.

V. Postoperative Procedures

A. It is important to record information regarding the sedation procedure in the patient's file just as you would document delivering local anesthesia or performing an operative procedure. Careful and thorough documentation is necessary for each patient. A later section of this chapter provides details of record-keeping procedures.

B. Turn off the unit using the master switch on the flowmeter.

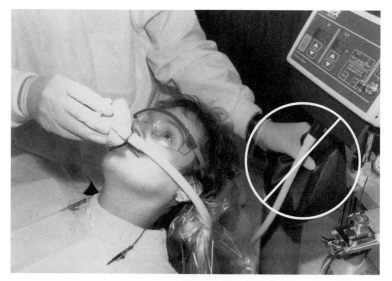

Figure 13-21   Do not purge the contents of the reservoir bag before postoperative oxygenation; this contaminates the operator's breathing zone unnecessarily.

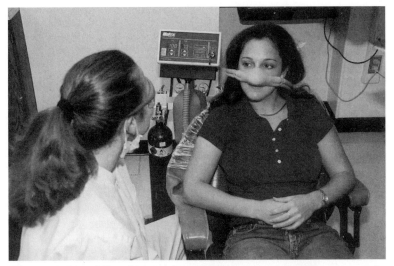

Figure 13-22   Offer additional minutes of oxygen until complete recovery is ensured.

Figure 13-23   Obtain postoperative vital sign measurements to assess recovery.

C. Turn off gas cylinders on a portable unit immediately following use. Central system cylinders are commonly turned off at the end of the day.
   1. Bleeding the lines on the portable unit at the end of the day purges the gas left in the lines into the ambient air.
   2. The amount, most likely, will be minimal; however, it is unnecessary contamination.

Figure 13-24   Dismiss patient when recovery is complete.

VI. Sterilization and Disinfection

A. Consult the manufacturer's instructions for best results regarding the sterilization and disinfection of specific sedation equipment. All team members that have contact with a patient or the sedation equipment should follow the guidelines for hand hygiene as outlined by the Centers for Disease Control and Prevention (Appendix G).

B. The level of disinfection and/or sterilization depends largely on the piece of equipment itself and its relation to patient contact or the contaminated environment.

1. As aforementioned, a clear bag barrier may be placed over the flowmeter as a means of protection against aerosols and splatter (Figure 13-25). If a bag barrier is not used, surface disinfection may be accomplished using a product similar to that used on other operatory surfaces (Figure 13-26).

2. The inside of the reservoir bag is only exposed to fresh gas. Therefore the inside does not have to be either disinfected or sterilized. However, the outside of the bag may be exposed to aerosols and splatter during operative procedures and should be, at least, disinfected.

Figure 13-25 Bag barriers may be used to protect equipment during procedures.

Figure 13-26 Surface disinfection of sedation equipment.

   a. Some reservoir bags are autoclavable whereas others will not stand the rigors of sterilization well. If you choose to sterilize a bag that is not specifically identified as being autoclavable, it is important to know that it will not last very long. A replacement bag should be readily available.

   b. Surface disinfection over time will also decrease the longevity of the bag. Check it frequently for leaks and always have a replacement bag on hand.

3. The conduction tubing is exposed to both the patient and the environment. There are no studies that verify disease transmission between patients through conduction tubing.

   a. The majority of the conduction tubing is able to withstand sterilization. However, if the tubing has a portion that is larger in diameter and corrugated, this piece is not able to withstand heat and will melt. This portion is typically the piece that comes off of the flowmeter and is where the fresh gas first enters the tubing. This section may be disinfected with a surface agent or covered with a barrier.

   b. The other portion of the conduction tubing may be sterilized. If the system has a plastic gauge that monitors the flow of the suction at the end of the hose, this piece may not be sterilized. It may be surface disinfected (Figure 13-27).

4. A laboratory study done in the late 1970s found that nasal bacteria could be transferred into the nasal hood.[3] There are two types of nasal hoods available: sterilizable and single-patient use.

   a. Autoclavable nasal hoods are available from all companies. Autoclavable hoods may contain latex or be latex-free. Sterilization of these products is recommended between patients.

   b. Nasal hoods that are designed for single-patient use are not autoclavable. They may be disposed of (Figure 13-28) or can be retained by the patient or office for a subsequent visit.

VII. Prudent Recordkeeping Procedures

A. Importance

1. The primary purpose for keeping accurate and complete records in a healthcare setting is to provide a written history of patient-operator interactions. This runs the gamut—from the patient's health history, medications, and chief concerns to treatment options, completed procedures, recommendations, and much more.

2. This history gives an account for future reference to yourself or others so that the patient receives continuity of care.

3. It is also a written record of chronologic events and experiences, making it a medicolegal document able to be used for you or against you in a court of law.

4. It is recommended that the person making an entry in a patient's record sign or initial the entry. This will hold all individuals accountable for the information, or lack thereof, that is written or unwritten.

Figure 13-27   Remove metal or plastic connections before sterilizing conduction tubing.

B. Completing the N_2O/O_2 sedation record
  1. Specific information obtained during N_2O/O_2 sedation should be recorded in the patient's file. This information may be recorded as part of the appointment entry on the patient's service record or on a separate form. Box 13-4 lists the items to include in the patient's file for each experience.
  2. If a separate form is used, it must be permanently attached to the patient's file. A new form is to be used for each experience (Figure 13-29).
  3. An example of an N_2O/O_2 sedation record can be found in Appendix C. It may be photocopied for office use.

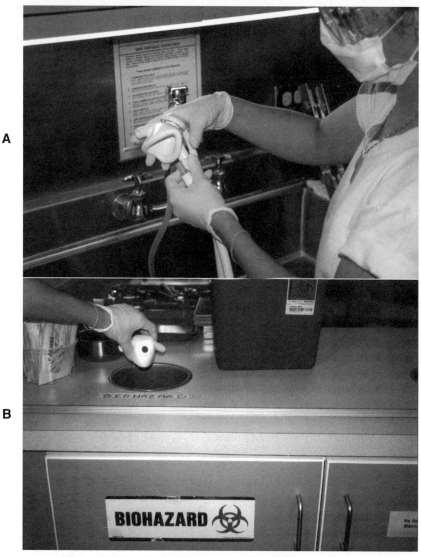

Figure 13-28 Single-patient use nasal hoods are not autoclavable.

BOX 13-4
Components of Sedation Record

Patient's name and date
ASA classification
Indications for N_2O/O_2 use
Preoperative, intraoperative, and postoperative vital sign values
Patient's tidal volume
Peak percentage of N_2O administered
Assessment of recovery (i.e., postoperative oxygenation time in minutes, patient responses to questions)
Adverse reactions and comments
Practitioner's signature or initials

```
┌─────────────────────────────────────────────────────────────────────┐
│                        N₂O/O₂ Sedation Record                        │
│                                                                       │
│   Date: 11-15-02    Patient Name: John Doe          Age: 42          │
│                                                                       │
│   ASA Classification:    I  ⓘⓘ  III  IV                               │
│   Indications for N₂O/O₂: mild anxiety, hypersensitive gag reflex    │
│   Procedural Data:        Preoperative   Intraoperative  Postoperative│
│                                          (moderate sedation)          │
│      Blood pressure:        140/86                         138/84     │
│      Pulse:                   76                             72       │
│      Respiration:             16                            16        │
│      SpO₂ (moderate sedation): ____                                   │
│                                                                       │
│      Tidal volume (L/min):  8.0      Peak % N₂O adm: 40%             │
│      Postop 100% O₂:         5     minutes                            │
│      Recovery (pt comments): " feel fine "                           │
│                                                                       │
│   Adverse Reactions/Comments:    Clinician's signature: QJohnson     │
│      Appt went well                                                   │
└─────────────────────────────────────────────────────────────────────┘
```

Figure 13-29   Sample completed sedation record.

REFERENCES

1. Malamed SF: *Sedation: a guide to patient management*, ed 4, St Louis, 2003, Mosby.
2. American Dental Association Council on Scientific Affairs: Nitrous oxide in the dental office, *J Am Dent Assoc* 128:364, 1997.
3. Hunt LM, Yagiela JA: Bacterial contamination and transmission by nitrous oxide sedation apparatus, *Oral Surg* 44(3):367,1977.

14
Recovery from N_2O/O_2 Sedation

Recovery from N_2O/O_2 sedation is an important part of the sedation experience. There are several aspects to complete recovery from the drug. The literature holds a plethora of references regarding psychologic and psychomotor effects that occur during N_2O/O_2 administration.[1-10] The extent of psychologic and psychomotor effects during N_2O/O_2 sedation is not the same for any two individuals. It can also be surmised from the literature that time for complete recovery from these effects cannot be reliably assessed.[1-10] Return to physiologic normalcy from N_2O/O_2 sedation appears to be readily apparent; however, the prudent practitioner acknowledges the potential for individual biovariability regarding all aspects of recovery and acts with common sense regarding patient dismissal from the clinical setting.

I. Principles of Recovery

A. Generally, emergence (recovery) is a mirror image of induction.[11] This mirror image includes patients returning to their original emotional state, as well as recovering from the pharmacologic action of the drug. N_2O evokes a rapid onset of clinical activity and thus a correlated rapid emergence from the sedation endpoint. Therefore, providing a calm, tranquil preoperative environment facilitates the sedative experience from beginning to end.

B. Physiologically, recovery occurs the same way for any individual. N_2O, as mentioned earlier, is principally exhaled unchanged from the lungs. However, the potential exists for postoperative symptoms such as lethargy, headache, and nausea to occur. Although opinions vary among researchers as to what causes these symptoms, we believe that postoperative oxygenation is required. Postoperative oxygenation remains an extremely important concept of recovery. Postoperatively, 100% O_2 must be administered for a minimum of 5 minutes. Depending on individual biovariability, this postoperative oxygenation period may be extended until both patient and operator are satisfied that adequate recovery has been achieved.

II. Psychologic and Psychomotor Effects

A. Investigation of effects. Several studies have been completed by reputable professionals investigating the effects of N_2O on psychomotor ability, memory, mood, and cognition.[1-10] Many tests have been commonly used to assess these functions: visual analog scales have been used to assess mood; psychomotor impairment has been assessed using digit-symbol substitution tests, paper-pencil tests, eye-hand coordination tests, automobile driving simulation, etc.; questionnaires have been used to ascertain degrees of euphoria, concentration, and attention. Results of these tests vary; however, experts agree that mental and psychomotor impairment does occur with N_2O, as it does with almost every other drug.

B. Psychologic and psychomotor impairment during N_2O/O_2 administration has been well established. Operators need to be assured to the greatest extent possible that patients are adequately recovered from sedation so they do not harm themselves or others upon dismissal from practitioners' offices. To date there are no references to cases in which patients who were dismissed after N_2O/O_2 sedation harmed or injured themselves or others because of incomplete recovery from the drug.

III. Technique for Assessing Adequate Recovery

A. Patient escorts. It is important to remember that not all patients recover to the extent that they may be dismissed without an escort. Depending on the circumstances of the situation, an educated practitioner must make this decision based on knowledge of the drug effects and the patient.

B. Assessment of a patient's response to questioning is subjective but in most cases valid.

   1. After the required postoperative oxygenation period of 5 minutes minimum, you should begin questioning patients about how they feel. Patients should indicate that they are feeling relaxed but not drowsy, lightheaded, groggy, dizzy, nauseous, etc.

   2. If there is any indication that a patient does not feel normal, assume that recovery is not complete. Additional postoperative oxygen time is required and continued until all responses are positive and indicative of normal feelings (Box 14-1).

C. Postoperative vital sign values are an objective measure of recovery.

   1. Generally, blood pressure values within 10 mm Hg (both systolic and diastolic) from preoperative readings are considered to be within an accepted comparable range.

   2. Likewise, postoperative pulse rate within 10 beats and respiration rate within 5 breaths are acceptable parameters for comparison (Figure 14-1).

   3. As mentioned earlier, a pulse oximeter can be used for obtaining and recording this information. Some machines produce a paper printout that can be attached to the patient's record for documentation purposes.

BOX 14-1

Assessing Recovery

Assessment begins following initial 5-minute postoperative oxygenation period
Obtain postoperative vital sign values
Question patient without removing O_2 for indications of:
Lethargy
Headache
Dizziness
Confusion
Nausea
If any symptoms present, continue O_2
Dismiss only when assured patient is fully recovered
Recommend escort if necessary

D. Psychomotor recovery from inhalation sedation has been addressed in the literature.

1. Early studies[12-14] recommended preoperative and postoperative drawing tests to determine visual-motor coordination and recovery. In the studies, recovery was complete within 3 to 5 minutes after termination of the N_2O.[12-14]

2. Jastak and Orendurff[15] investigated psychomotor recovery by using a driving simulation test. Participants were evaluated for errors in steering, braking, signaling, and speeding. All postsedation figures correlated with presedation values, thereby concluding that patients could safely operate a motor vehicle after N_2O/O_2 sedation.[15] This study has been the foundation for practitioners dismissing patients without an escort. Recently, Martin et al[16] confirms the claim that driving ability is not impaired following flexible sigmoidoscopy screening using N_2O.

3. There is a simple hand-eye coordination exercise that can be done in the office to assess psychomotor recovery. Have patients extend an arm out to

Figure 14-1 Obtain postoperative vital sign values to assist assessment of recovery.

the side; then give instructions to place their little finger on the tip of their nose. The exercise may be done with either or both hands. Accuracy is subjective; however, if this simple skill cannot be completed, it may be necessary to reevaluate adequate recovery.

IV. Guidelines for Patient Discharge Following Moderate Sedation According to the ASA Practice Guidelines for Sedation and Analgesia by Non-Anesthesiologists

A. Patients should be alert and oriented; infants and patients whose mental status was initially abnormal should have returned to their baseline status. Practitioners and parents must be aware that pediatric patients are at risk for airway obstruction should the head fall forward while the child is secured in a car seat.
B. Vital sign values should be stable and within acceptable limits.
C. Use of scoring systems may assist in documentation of fitness for discharge.
D. Outpatients and their escorts should be provided with written instructions regarding postprocedure diet, medications, activities, and a telephone number to be called in case of emergency.[17] (Remember, patients who are minimally sedated *do not typically require* escorts.)
E. Documentation of adequate recovery must be maintained for each patient visit.[17]

V. Recovery Time

A. Recovery time has continued to be a subject of research studies through the years. There are a wide variety of recommendations regarding the number of minutes it takes for complete recovery following sedation with N$_2$O. The important factor to remember is that each patient is different and recovery times may vary.[18-20] *Ultimately, responsibility lies in the hands of the operator to make an educated decision as to the complete recovery of patients before their dismissal* (Figure 14-2).

REFERENCES
1. Cheam EW et al: The effect of nitrous oxide on the performance of psychomotor tests: a dose-response study, *Anaesthesia* 50:764, 1995.
2. Fagan D et al: A dose-response study of the effects of inhaled nitrous oxide on psychological performance and mood, *Psychopharmacology* 116:333, 1994.
3. Dohrn CS et al: Subjective and psychomotor effects of nitrous oxide in healthy volunteers, *Behav Pharmacol* 3:19, 1992.
4. Armstrong PJ et al: Effects of nitrous oxide on psychological performance: a dose-response study using inhalation of concentrations up to 15%, *Psychopharmacology* 117:486, 1995.
5. Zacny JP et al: Time course of effects of brief inhalations of nitrous oxide in normal volunteers, *Addiction* 89:831, 1994.
6. Zacny JP et al: The subjective, behavioral and cognitive effects of subanesthetic concentrations of isoflurane and nitrous oxide in healthy volunteers, *Psychopharmacology* 114:409, 1994.

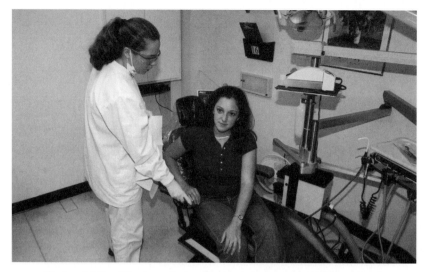

Figure 14-2   Dismiss patient only when adequate recovery is achieved.

7. Yajnik S et al: Effects of marijuana history on the subjective, psychomotor, and reinforcing effects of nitrous oxide in humans, *Drug Alcohol Depend* 36:227, 1994.
8. Tiplady R, Sinclair WA, Morrison LM: Effects of nitrous oxide on psychological performance, *Psychopharmacol Bull* 28:207, 1992.
9. Ramsay JS et al: Paradoxical effects of nitrous oxide on human memory, *Psychopharmacology* 106:370, 1992.
10. Thompson JM et al: Cognitive properties of sedation agents: comparison of the effects of nitrous oxide and midazolam on memory and mood, *Br Dent J* 187(10): 557, 1999.
11. Eger EI II: Uptake and distribution. In Miller RD, editor: *Anesthesia*, vol 1, ed 4, New York, 1994, Churchill Livingstone.
12. Newman MG, Trieger N, Miller JC: Measuring recovery from anesthesia: a simple test, *Anesth Anal* 48:136, 1969.
13. Trieger N, Newman MG, Miller JC: An objective measure of recovery, *Anesth Prog* 16:4, 1969.
14. Trieger N et al: Nitrous oxide: a study of physiological and psychomotor effects, *J Am Dent Assoc* 82:142, 1971.
15. Jastak JT, Orendurff D: Recovery from nitrous sedation, *Anesth Prog* 22:113, 1975.
16. Martin JP et al: Inhaled patient-administered nitrous oxide/oxygen mixture does not impair driving ability when used as analgesia during screening flexible sigmoidoscopy, *Gastrointest Endosc* 51(6):701, 2000.
17. American Dental Association: *Guidelines for the use of conscious sedation, deep sedation and general anesthesia for dentists*, Chicago, 2002, American Dental Association.
18. McKercher TC et al: Recovery and enhancement of reflex reaction time after nitrous oxide analgesia, *JADA* 101:785, 1980.
19. Korttila K et al: Time course of mental and psychomotor effects of 30 percent nitrous oxide during inhalation and recovery, *Anesthesiology* 54:220, 1981.
20. Trojan J et al: Immediate recovery of psychomotor function after patient-administered nitrous oxide/oxygen inhalation for colonoscopy, *Endoscopy* 29:17, 1997.

15

Multidisciplinary Application of N_2O/O_2 Sedation

Some health disciplines have been using N_2O/O_2 sedation for mild-to-moderate pain control and anxiety relief for many years. Other healthcare professionals have recently revisited its use, not as a general anesthetic, but as an effective analgesic-sedative for the many ambulatory and outpatient procedures being performed today.

Articles referring to N_2O/O_2 sedation in obstetrics are found in the literature because of long-standing use in Great Britain and the United States.[1] Emergency care personnel, in both the field and the hospital setting, have also been long-term providers of this therapy.[2] Other disciplines have limited literature citations.

N_2O may have broad applicability in an era in which greater numbers of surgical procedures are being performed in outpatient settings. N_2O/O_2 sedation is a viable treatment alternative for outpatient procedures regardless of discipline.

I. Emergency Medicine

A. Prehospital care in the ambulance
   1. An analgesic agent appropriate for prehospital emergency pain control should possess several specific characteristics. Properties that are desirable are rapid onset of clinical action, no effect on level of consciousness, no significant side effects, and no masking of other conditions, which would ultimately interfere with the diagnostic evaluation at the hospital.
   2. N_2O possesses many of these characteristics. Several researchers support the notion that N_2O possesses many of these ideal characteristics necessary in this discipline.[3-5]
B. Historical use of N_2O/O_2 in emergency medicine
   1. The first self-administered, fixed-ratio system used in an ambulance service was implemented by Peter Baskett, from England, in 1969. A mixture of 50% N_2O and 50% O_2 was delivered to the patient using an on-demand system. His idea was that patients in an ambulatory situation should control their own sedation by self-administering this fixed-ratio mixture of gases. Baskett concluded his clinical trials (305 patients with significant decrease in pain and no serious complications) with the claim that N_2O/O_2 was safe and effective for use in emergency medicine.[2]

2. Not long after the initiation of this type of sedation in England, health-care providers in the United States began using it for emergency medicine. In 1979, Flomenbaum et al[6] were the first to promote its use in United States emergency departments and to document such use in the literature.

C. Current usage and effectiveness statistics

1. Recently emergency medical services (EMS) have placed priority on early patient stabilization, safe transportation, and effective communication systems (Figure 15-1). Great strides have been made in these areas, making services to the public safer and more effective. Pain control has always been a focus and is gaining greater attention. The issues of masking symptoms or making conditions worse before hospital access are important considerations in the decision to attend to pain with an analgesic agent.

2. EMS personnel continue to use Baskett's fixed-ratio, self-administration technique. This technique is popular because of its portability in the field. Emergency departments in hospital settings may use the fixed-ratio, on-demand equipment or they may use continuous-flow machines like those that have been used in dentistry.

3. Researchers have cited many instances of successful uses of N_2O/O_2 in the prehospital and emergency department settings. Gamis, Knapp, and Glenski[7] completed a study using N_2O/O_2 on pediatric patients requiring laceration repair in the emergency department at Children's Mercy Hospital in Kansas City, Missouri. Thirty-four children participated and were placed in either a treatment group that used a ratio of 30% N_2O and 70% O_2 or a control group using 100% O_2. A clinically significant difference was found in the pain scores between groups of children older than

Figure 15-1   Stabilizing the patient at the scene. (From Stoy: *Mosby's first responder textbook*, St. Louis, 1997, Mosby.)

8 years. Although no statistically significant difference was found with children in the 2 to 7 age group, pain scores decreased when N$_2$O/O$_2$ was used.[7] In another study, N$_2$O/O$_2$ provided a significant reduction in pain and anxiety during venous cannulation in an emergency department.[8]

    4. White et al[9] recently confirmed that prehospital pain control can be improved especially for patients with suspected extremity fractures. They acknowledge N$_2$O as a viable option.

D. Indications for use of N$_2$O/O$_2$ in emergency medicine

    1. Many uses have been described in the literature.[3-5,10,11] Examples of procedures in which N$_2$O/O$_2$ has been used for musculoskeletal injuries include fractures, strains and sprains, and dislocations.

    2. When providing patient care of the skin, N$_2$O/O$_2$ may be used when placing and removing sutures; incising abscesses; removing cysts, nevi, or warts; débriding wounds; and dressing burns.

    3. Head injuries that are nonneurologic in origin may be successfully treated with N$_2$O/O$_2$. Examples are abrasion debridement, removing or draining abscesses or cysts, removing foreign objects from ears, and removing or replacing teeth after trauma.

    4. Examples of other procedures include removing or changing drains, catheterization, biopsies, hemorrhoid removal, splinting, extrications, and complicated transfer or movement of patients.

E. Contraindications for use of N$_2$O/O$_2$ in emergency medicine

    1. In emergency cases in which pneumothorax or a closed head injury is suspected, N$_2$O is not recommended.[10]

F. Equipment

    1. The equipment used in ambulances consists of the gas mixture stored in either a single cylinder or in separate tanks. In some countries the single-cylinder system is preferred because it is lightweight and easy to operate. A major disadvantage of this 50:50 mixture is the instability of the gases in one cylinder. If the temperature of the mixture is allowed to fall below 5.5° C for even a minimal amount of time, the N$_2$O separates and settles to the bottom of the cylinder. A high concentration of O$_2$ could be dispensed under these conditions, which would mean that pure N$_2$O would be dispensed as the O$_2$ is depleted.

    2. To date, the United States has not approved the single-cylinder system for use because of the potential for 100% N$_2$O to be delivered. However, this system is popular in countries such as the United Kingdom, Canada, Australia, and New Zealand.

    3. The Matrx Medical Company offers the safety of a double-tank system and the portability of the single-cylinder system. Its major advantage is that it weighs only 11 pounds and can be carried over the shoulder or harnessed to the back. The Nitronox field model is shown in Figure 15-2.

    4. In the field setting, patients are required to hold a mask and place it over their mouth and nose to inspire the analgesic. If the patient is unable to hold the mask because of an injury, a mouthpiece can be held tight between the lips and teeth, allowing for inspiration through the mouth.

Figure 15-2   Nitronox field model. (Courtesy Matrx Medical Inc., Orchard Park, New York.)

G. Products
1. The 50:50 gas mixture that is primarily used in the United Kingdom, Canada, and Australia is called Entonox. It is manufactured by several companies.
2. Nitronox is available both in the United States and abroad.

II. Obstetrics and Gynecology

A. Labor and delivery
1. The literature is saturated with studies reporting manageable, successful labor and deliveries using N_2O/O_2 therapy.
2. A Russian physician began using N_2O/O_2 in 1880 as an analgesic during labor. His experiments led him to the conclusion that it relieved labor pain without harming mother or baby.[12]
3. Swedish literature citations confirm the safety record of N_2O anesthesia. Records show no reproductive problems in nearly 300 women exposed to N_2O.[13]
4. A 1981 hospital study in Wales evaluated the effectiveness of Entonox delivered through a nasal catheter to women in labor. Both midwives and mothers agreed that Entonox provided labor pain relief.[14] Administration by nasal catheter was comfortable and nonintrusive; however, this method of delivery should not be used because of environmental contamination.

5. A 1994 study in Toronto done by Carstoniu, Levytam, and Norman[15] raised questions about the validity and reliability of previous research on N_2O/O_2 use in labor, citing methodologic flaws as the primary weakness of early research. In the study, relief of pain and oxygen saturation were the foci. Results showed no statistical difference when patients used N_2O/O_2 or compressed air. Patients did recognize the difference in gases, and when offered to continue either, they preferred N_2O/O_2. The oxygen desaturation factor was insignificant, and authors indicated O_2 levels were enhanced between contractions.[15]

B. Gynecologic laparoscopy
1. Although CO_2 is used traditionally as the insufflation gas for laparoscopy, N_2O may be used as part of a combination technique.
2. The American Association of Gynecologic Laparoscopists stated that no adverse incidents occurred in more than 20,000 procedures when N_2O/O_2 was used in some capacity.[16]

III. Dermatology

A. Hair transplantation
1. Hair transplantation is cited as a procedure in which N_2O/O_2 can provide satisfactory analgesia without negatively affecting patient cooperation or producing untoward side effects. Patients in a study by Sadick and Militana[17] responded overwhelmingly (94%) that they preferred N_2O/O_2 over 10 mg diazepam (Valium) and the Dermajet method of lidocaine delivery. Because this surgery requires repeated injections of local anesthetic, the sedative nature of N_2O/O_2 allows for increased patient tolerance.
2. An N_2O/O_2 advantage noted in hair transplantation is the rapid elimination of the drug versus others, such as diazepam, which has a much longer latent period without reversal.[17]

B. Skin treatments and cancer surgeries. Chemical peeling and skin cancer surgeries are also mentioned in the literature as being facilitated by N_2O/O_2 sedation.[17,18]

C. Liposuction
1. Liposuction has become a popular procedure. Local anesthetic infiltration has been combined with IM, IV, inhalation sedation, or general anesthesia for this procedure. Professionals state that although many drugs interact with local anesthetics required by this procedure, N_2O/O_2 does not.
2. Dermatologists' experience with N_2O/O_2 is minimal; however, they support its adjunctive properties to local anesthetics.[19] Maloney, Coleman, and Mora[20] concur with others in the dermatology field who support the use of N_2O/O_2. In their study, 46 of 47 patients indicated that they would request N_2O/O_2 for future visits and thought it should be used more in the discipline.

IV. Podiatry

A. Ambulatory foot surgeries
   1. Ambulatory foot surgery was successfully accomplished in 1966. It was the first mention in the literature of N_2O/O_2 use in this discipline.[21]
B. Various other podiatric procedures
   1. In a 1972 study, Mosher and Sorkin[22] provided descriptive evidence of 21 patients requiring varying podiatric procedures while receiving N_2O/O_2 titrated to appropriate levels. No significant side effects were noted; amnesia was reported in 19% of patients. All patients indicated a relaxed sense of well-being. Several advantages of N_2O/O_2 analgesia were listed, one of which was the enhancement of local anesthetic effects.
   2. Some of the procedures reported being performed using N_2O/O_2 are digital arthroplasty, nail matricectomy, subungual exostectomy, bunionectomy, excision of digital mass, digital arthrodesis, excision of hallux ossicle, Tailor's bunionectomy, syndactylia, and excision of plantar mass.[22]
C. Use with diazepam (Valium). Another study (1982) encouraged specialists to use N_2O/O_2 concomitantly with 10 mg of diazepam. The authors stated success in more than 150 cases. Their attitude regarding this technique is professed as "a new era in the attainment of near-painless podiatric surgery."[23]

V. Ophthalmology

A. Eye surgery
   1. The most common anesthetic techniques involve IV sedation and retrobulbar block or topical anesthesia only. Cataract surgery using N_2O/O_2 sedation is referenced in the journal *Ophthalmic Surgery*.[24]
   2. N_2O/O_2 can be used instead of IM premedication to prepare patients for the necessary local anesthetic placement. McMahan[24] used N_2O/O_2 therapy on 800 patients for cataract surgery with great success.
B. Implant surgery
   1. Implant surgery performed at the Hawaiian Eye Surgicenter includes N_2O/O_2 as part of the procedure. Clinicians there wanted an analgesic-sedative for assistance during the local injection but did not want the prolonged effects of other drugs. They wanted patients to be fully recovered for prompt dismissal.
   2. Clinicians expressed satisfaction with the calming, amnestic effects with their 50% N_2O and 50% O_2 technique.[25]
C. Ambulatory setting. Specialists in the ophthalmology discipline acknowledge interest in the use of N_2O/O_2 sedation in the ambulatory setting.[26]

VI. Cryosurgery

A. In cryosurgery, rather than being used for its amnestic effects, N_2O is used to cool metal instruments, which in turn initiates the freezing or tissue necrosis of a lesion.
B. N_2O is preferred over liquid nitrogen because it is easier to handle.[27]
C. Successful management of obstructive malignant airway lesions and early superficial lung cancer using bronchoscopic cryotherapy was shown by Noppen et al[28] in Belgium.

VII. Psychiatry and Psychology

A. Depression
   1. N_2O/O_2 has been used for patients exhibiting chronic anxiety. Depressed patients have found relief from N_2O/O_2 therapy.
   2. In an early study, N_2O was found to be more effective than thiopental with electroconvulsive therapy for treatment of depression.[29] However, methohexital or propofol plus succinylcholine are still most commonly used.
B. Schizophrenia
   1. Traditionally, using N_2O/O_2 with schizophrenic patients has been cautioned because of individual biovariability and the potential for provoking their psychoses.
   2. Gillman[30] found three of four patients became relaxed after N_2O/O_2 use. He documented problems with one patient.
C. Sex research. Sex research has included N_2O/O_2 therapy as well. Research done by Gillman and Lichtigfeld[31] shows females unable to achieve orgasm became multiorgasmic with therapy that included N_2O/O_2.
D. Hyperactivity
   1. deWet et al[34] have also used N_2O as a possible treatment modality for hyperactivity. They report a 50% positive response rate and intend to continue with further controlled studies.

VIII. Endoscopy

A. Gastrointestinal endoscopy
   1. Diehl et al[35] presented N_2O/O_2 research results at the American Society of Gastrointestinal Endoscopy (ASGE) 1996 annual session. They indicated success with N_2O/O_2 in the outpatient setting at significantly less cost. In addition, patients generally accepted the procedure and clinicians felt that administering N_2O/O_2 was not problematic and appreciated patient tolerance. The study also looked at differences between using N_2O/O_2 or IV-infused barbiturates. No statistically significant differences were found.[35] Forbes and Collins[36] compared N_2O/O_2 to conventional intravenous seda-

tion for colonoscopy in 2000. They concluded that this may be a viable option for some patients and reported the advantage of faster recovery.
B. These initial results have been met with enthusiasm by a number of specialists in the field of endoscopy. This research may open a new vista in endoscopy.

IX. Addiction Withdrawal

A. Pentazocine (Talwin)
   1. N_2O has been investigated as a potential therapeutic drug for addiction withdrawal of certain substances. Kripke and Hechtman[37] were the first to mention this innovation in 1972 when treating pentazocine addiction. Pentazocine is a narcotico-analog analgesic. It is contraindicated for treating patients using narcotics.
   2. Pentazocine was used in significant amounts to obviate the continual severe pain of an esophageal (potash) injury plaguing a 14-year-old girl. The patient became addicted to the drug, and clinicians used N_2O/O_2 to wean her from it. Advantages of this therapy were the freedom from pain and the ease of delivery at her home.[37]
B. Alcohol
   1. Lichtigfeld and Gillman[38] found N_2O/O_2 to be effective for alcohol withdrawal in more than 5000 cases in South Africa.
   2. A single 20-minute application of analgesic N_2O/O_2 to a patient during admittance to a treatment center relieves initial withdrawal symptoms without causing significant sedation, which allows for other social detoxification therapies to be initiated immediately.[38] Gillman and Lichtigfeld[39] report 90% of acute alcoholic withdrawal states were reversed within the first 60 minutes of a single dose treatment of N_2O/O_2. Other discoveries made using N_2O/O_2 included reduced hospital stays and decreased doses of other medications with no addictive propensity to N_2O.[40]
C. Nicotine and marijuana addiction. N_2O/O_2 sedation has also been experimented with successfully in treating nicotine and marijuana addiction.[40]

X. Radiology

A. Painful procedures
   1. Analgesic-anxiolytic N_2O/O_2 has proved beneficial in the discipline of radiology.
   2. In a study on radiologic procedures, 50 of 53 patients reported that N_2O/O_2 sedation improved their procedures. Some of the procedures in which N_2O/O_2 sedation may be appropriate are aortoperipheral arteriography, percutaneous biopsies, visceral arteriography, percutaneous cholangiography, biliary catheter placement, biliary stone retrieval, bilateral ureterastent placement, hepatic artery catheter placement, liver abscess drainage, and bilateral temporomandibular joint arthroscopy.[41] Patients using N_2O/O_2 sedation are far more cooperative when asked to remain still than patients using IV sedation.[41]

B. Magnetic resonance imaging (MRI)
1. The MRI procedure is often complicated or even contraindicated for patients who are claustrophobic. The procedure requires the patient to be confined to a small space and remain very still for an extended period.
2. Often patients require some type of sedation for anxiety management so that accuracy of the procedure is ensured. N$_2$O/O$_2$ sedation can be a viable option for this procedure. However, it may be necessary to explore ways to improve the accessibility of the delivery equipment within the spatial confines of the MRI equipment (Figure 15-3).

XI. Dentistry

A. Pain and anxiety
1. Although local anesthetics revolutionized pain control in dentistry, administering the anesthetic with a needle is still difficult for some patients to take.
2. Pain and fear are prohibiting factors for seeking dental treatment; more than 40% of the population avoids the dental office for these reasons.[42] N$_2$O/O$_2$ sedation offers a way to overcome these barriers.
B. Widespread use in the discipline
1. Dentistry has been and continues to be a significant supporter and proprietor of N$_2$O/O$_2$ sedation. It has been used for most procedures and by all specialties within the profession.

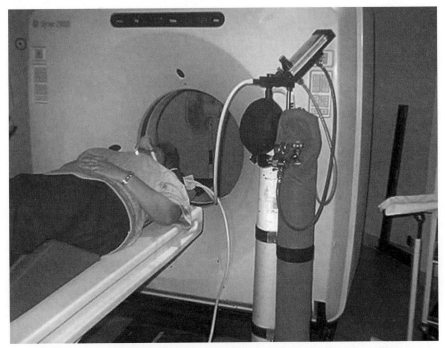

Figure 15-3 N$_2$O/O$_2$ administration during a radiologic procedure. (Photo courtesy Dr. Carlos Plateroti, Buenos Aires, Argentina.)

2. The dental profession uses N_2O/O_2 sedation for procedures in the areas of periodontics, prosthodontics, orthodontics, dental hygiene, restorative dentistry, oral and maxillofacial surgery, endodontics, geriatrics, and especially pedodontics.[43]

C. Depression of the gag reflex. A recent study documents that N_2O/O_2 sedation works well to depress a hypersensitive gag reflex, which can be problematic during dental procedures.[44]

XII. Pediatrics

A. Painful and anxiety-producing situations
1. Pediatric patients present special concerns for healthcare professionals. The more positive healthcare experiences children have, the more likely that they will behave positively during future visits. Also, repeated positive childhood experiences create positive adult attitudes and behaviors. Think of the number of adult patients that are anxious because of a bad childhood experience.
2. In spite of a trusting, caring, and kind relationship between a healthcare worker and a child, some procedures hurt. No matter how the clinician prepares children psychologically for pain, the actual stick with the needle is what they remember. In dentistry, N_2O/O_2 sedation of children has been successful for many years. It is estimated that 88% of pediatric dentists use this method of sedation in their practices.[45]
3. Over a 9-year period Griffin, Campbell, and Jones[46] researched the effect of N_2O/O_2 sedation on more than 3000 children and teenagers for minor surgical procedures. The procedures included laceration or fracture repair, nevi excision, wart removal, abscess incision, and removal of items such as slivers, needles, nails, and fishhooks. Ninety-nine percent of the patients indicated that they would choose to have N_2O/O_2 sedation at a future visit.

B. Amnestic and hypnosuggestive properties
1. These properties are advantageous when treating children. The short attention span of a child often requires additional patient management and time when completing a procedure. The relaxed patient and altered perception of time offered by N_2O/O_2 sedation greatly assists the practitioner.
2. Children are much more hypnosuggestive by nature than adults. A calm, slow, soothing voice facilitates the action of N_2O/O_2 immensely. See Chapter 16 for information specific to pediatrics.

XIII. Acute Myocardial Infarction

A. Reduced pain and anxiety
1. Analgesic levels of N_2O/O_2 have been successfully implemented to relieve acute pain during myocardial infarction (MI). The pathophysio-

logic process of an MI results in extreme pain and typically includes tremendous anxiety.

2. Several studies conducted from 1962 to 1965 in the former Soviet Republic proved the effectiveness of N_2O/O_2 with MI.[47,48] Its use in the United States at that time is documented in the literature as well.[11,49] Results of research by Thompson and Lown[50] indicate some relief of pain in 74% of patients. Patients with mild pain were more likely to get significant relief than those experiencing moderate-to-agonizing pain. In those cases, narcotics provided adjuvant analgesic therapy.[50]

3. Currently, the most common pain relief protocols for acute MI include nitroglycerin, beta blockers, and morphine.

B. Supplemental oxygen

1. N_2O/O_2 proved beneficial for those patients being treated in an ambulatory setting for coronary artery disease by enriching the O_2 supply to the heart.[4]

2. Although the O_2 is critical to the myocardium, the N_2O works as the analgesic-sedative for the patient.[4,9,50]

XIV. Terminally Ill Patients

A. Cancer or terminal illness

1. Patients with cancer or in terminal stages of illness often have unbearable pain.[51]

2. In such cases the issue of adequate pain control is a primary focus of the patient's family and significant others. They want their loved one to be comfortable in the final stages of life or when suffering a debilitating illness.

B. Quality of life

1. Fosburg and Crone[52] report that some patients continue IV-infused narcotics in conjunction with N_2O/O_2 treatment, whereas others prefer N_2O/O_2 alone. Keating and Kundrat[53] report that 81% of N_2O treatments provided improvement in pain that lasted from 30 minutes to 2 hours. In addition, they report increased activity, smiling, and communicability in patients.

2. Patients may be treated at home with N_2O/O_2 therapy and can often control their own therapy. In many instances of terminal illness, the N_2O/O_2 therapy improved patients' moods and appetites, and patients communicated more freely.

C. Hemodynamics

1. The hemodynamic issues surrounding continuous, long-term use of N_2O/O_2 are obviously not as important as relief of pain and anxiety for these patients in final stages of life.

2. Again, patient comfort is a top priority; restful, relaxed, pain-free last days are intensely sought by all terminally ill patients.

XV. Miscellaneous Procedures

A. Gillman and Lichtigfeld[40] cite that symptoms associated with various neurologic disorders have been eliminated with the use of N_2O/O_2 sedation. Some examples are Tourette's syndrome, neuroleptic-induced akathisia, and spasmodic torticollis. The article refers to these as preliminary investigations that require specific organized study.[40]

B. N_2O was shown to be an effective analgesic for patients undergoing percutaneous liver biopsy. Pain scores were significantly lower for patients in the N_2O/O_2 treatment group versus patients treated with a placebo. Investigators in this study cited several favorable characteristics of N_2O in addition to its analgesic potential.[54]

C. Migraine headaches have been treated with analgesic concentrations of N_2O/O_2. It seems the analgesic and sedative properties of N_2O/O_2 assist with the management of migraine symptoms.

1. In the literature, a 30-minute treatment of N_2O/O_2 titrated specifically to the patient's needs brought total relief within that period.[32] A more recent study validates this claim and indicates 80% of 22 patients with acute migraine symptoms who came to the emergency department did not require rescue medication following treatment with N_2O/O_2.[33]

REFERENCES

1. Minnett RJ: Self-administered anaesthesia in childbirth, *Br Med J* 1:501, 1934.
2. Baskett PJ, Withnell A: Use of Entonox on the ambulance service, *Br Med J* 2:41, 1970.
3. Stewart RD: Nitrous oxide sedation/analgesia in emergency medicine, *Ann Emerg Med* 14:139, 1985.
4. Amey BD, Ballinger JA, Harrison EE: Prehospital administration of nitrous oxide for control of pain, *Ann Emerg Med* 10:247, 1981.
5. Pons PT: Nitrous oxide analgesia, *Emerg Med Clin North Am* 6:777, 1988.
6. Flomenbaum N et al: Self-administered nitrous oxide: an adjunct analgesic, *J Am Col Emerg Phys* 8:95, 1979.
7. Gamis AS, Knapp JF, Glenski JA: Nitrous oxide analgesia in a pediatric emergency department, *Ann Emerg Med* 18:177, 1989.
8. Gerhardt RT et al: Inhaled nitrous oxide versus placebo as an analgesic and anxiolytic adjunct to peripheral intravenous cannulation, *Am J Emerg Med* 19(6):492, 2001.
9. White LJ et al: Prehospital use of analgesia for suspected extremity fractures, *Prehosp Emerg Care* 4(3):205, 2000.
10. Pinell MC, Linscott MS: Nitrous oxide in the emergency department, *Am J Emerg Med* 5:395, 1987.
11. Hayes GB: Relief of cardiac chest pain in the field, *Emerg Care Q* 3:49, 1987.
12. Marx GF, Katsnelson T: The introduction of nitrous oxide analgesia into obstetrics, *Obstet Gynecol* 80:715, 1992.
13. Santos AC, Pedersen H: Current controversies in obstetric anesthesia, *Anesth Anal* 78:753, 1994.
14. Arthurs GJ, Rosen M: Acceptability of continuous nasal nitrous oxide during labour: a field trial in six maternity hospitals, *Anaesthesia* 36:384, 1981.

15. Carstoniu J, Levytam S, Norman P: Nitrous oxide in early labor: safety and analgesic efficacy assessed by a double-blind, placebo-controlled study, *Anesthesiology* 80:30, 1994.

16. Ohlgisser M, Sorokin Y, Heifetz M: Gynecologic laparoscopy, *Obstet Gynecol Surv* 40:385, 1985.

17. Sadick NS, Militana CJ: Use of nitrous oxide in hair transplantation surgery, *J Dermatol Surg Oncol* 20:186, 1994.

18. Boullie MC: Nitrous oxide cryosurgery applied to skin cancers, *Dermatol Surg* 23(8):714, 1997.

19. Klein JA: Anesthesia for liposuction in dermatologic surgery, *J Dermatol Surg Oncol* 14:1124, 1988.

20. Maloney JM, Coleman WP, Mora R: Analgesia induced by nitrous oxide and oxygen as an adjunct to local anesthesia in dermatologic surgery, *J Dermatol Surg. Oncol* 6:939, 1980.

21. Arancia L: Nitrous oxide inhalation analgesia in ambulatory foot surgery, *J Am Coll Foot Surg* 5:111, 1966.

22. Mosher MR, Sorkin BS: Nitrous oxide/oxygen analgesia in podiatric surgery, *J Am Podiatry Assoc* 62:142, 1972.

23. Harris WC, Alpert WJ, Gill JJ: Nitrous oxide and valium use in podiatric surgery for production of conscious-sedation, *J Am Podiatry Assoc* 72:505, 1982.

24. McMahan LB: Nitrous oxide analgesia for cataract surgery, *Ophthalmic Surg* 13:307, 1982.

25. Corboy JM: Nitrous oxide analgesia for outpatient surgery, *Am Intra-Ocular Implant Soc J* 10:232, 1984.

26. Thompson V: Personal communication, September 1997.

27. Sullivan JH: Cryosurgery in ophthalmic practice, *Ophthalmic Surg* 10:37, 1979.

28. Noppen M et al: Bronchoscopic cryotherapy: preliminary experience, *Acta Clinical Belgica* 56(2):73, 2001.

29. Brill NW et al: Relative effectiveness of various forms of electroconvulsive therapy, *Arch Neurol Psychiatry* 81:109, 1959.

30. Gillman MA: Analgesic nitrous oxide as a therapeutic and investigative tool in neurological conditions. In Sinha KK, editor: *Progress in clinical neurosciences*, vol 2, Ranchi, 1985, Neurological Society of India.

31. Gillman MA, Lichtigfeld FJ: The effects of nitrous oxide and naloxone on orgasm in human females: a preliminary report, *J Sex Res* 19:49, 1986.

32. Stanley A: Migraine treated by inhalation sedation using nitrous oxide and oxygen, *Brit Dent J* 149:54, 1980.

33. Triner WR et al: Nitrous oxide for the treatment of acute migraine headache, *Am J Emerg Med* 17(3):252, 1999.

34. deWet J et al: Psychotropic analgesic nitrous oxide (PAN) for hyperactivity, *Aust N Z J Psychiatry* 35(4):543, 2001.

35. Diehl DL et al: Nitrous oxide (N$_2$O) vs intravenous sedation in upper gastrointestinal endoscopy (EGD): a prospective randomized controlled trial, *Gastrointest Endosc* 43:310, 1996.

36. Forbes GM, Collins BJ: Nitrous oxide for colonoscopy: a randomized controlled study, *Gastrointest Endosc* 51(3):271, 2000.

37. Kripke BJ, Hechtman HB: Nitrous oxide for pentazocine addiction and for intractable pain: report of case, *Anesth Analg* 51:520, 1972.

38. Lichtigfeld FJ, Gillman MA: The treatment of alcoholic withdrawal states with oxygen and nitrous oxide, *S Afr Med J* 61:349, 1982.

39. Gillman MA, Lichtigfeld FJ: Randomized double-blind trial of psychotropic analgesic nitrous oxide compared with diazepam for alcohol withdrawal state, *J Subst Abuse Treat* 22:129, 2002.
40. Gillman MA, Lichtigfeld FJ: Analgesic nitrous oxide in neuropsychiatry: past, present and future, *Intern J Neurosci* 49:75, 1989.
41. Katzen BT, Edwards KC: Nitrous-oxide analgesia for interventional radiologic procedures, *Am J Roentgenol* 140:145, 1983.
42. Ayer WA et al: Overcoming dental fear: strategies for its prevention and management, *J Am Dent Assoc* 107:18, 1983.
43. Malamed SF: *Sedation: a guide to patient management*, ed 4, St Louis, 2003, Mosby.
44. Chidiac JJ et al: Gagging prevention using nitrous oxide or table salt: a comparative pilot study, *Int J Prosth* 14(4):364, 2001.
45. Davis MJ: Conscious sedation practices in pediatric dentistry: a survey of members of the American Board of Pediatric Dentistry College of Diplomates, *Pediatr Dent* 10:328, 1988.
46. Griffin GC, Campbell VD, Jones R: Nitrous oxide-oxygen sedation for minor surgery, *J Am Med Assoc* 245:2411, 1981.
47. Iosava KV: Analgesic anesthesia with nitrous oxide in pain syndrome caused by coronary insufficiency (clinico-biochemical studies), *Kardiologiia* 5:54, 1965.
48. Pekker IL: Nitrous oxide anesthesia with pipolphan pre-medication in myocardial infarct at a first aid station, *Sov Med* 28:103, 1965.
49. Keer F et al: Nitrous oxide analgesia in myocardial infarction, *Lancet* 1:63, 1972.
50. Thompson PL, Lown B: Nitrous oxide as an analgesic in acute myocardial infarction, *J Am Med Assoc* 235:924, 1976.
51. Foley KM: The treatment of pain in the patient with cancer, *CA Cancer J Clin* 36:194, 1986.
52. Fosburg MT, Crone RK: Nitrous oxide analgesia for refractory pain in the terminally ill, *J Am Med Assoc* 250:511, 1983.
53. Keating HJ III, Kundrat M: Patient-controlled analgesia with nitrous oxide in cancer pain, *J Pain Symptom Manage* 11:126, 1996.
54. Brodsky JB: Toxicity of nitrous oxide. In Eger EI II, editor: *Nitrous oxide, N_2O*, New York, 1985, Elsevier Science Publishing.

SUGGESTED READINGS

Cruickshank JC, Sykes SH: Office sedation, *Adv Dermatol* 7:291, 1992.
Edwards FJ: The art of sedation in the emergency department, *J Am Acad Phys Assist* 7:128, 1994.
Henderson JM et al: Administration of nitrous oxide to pediatric patients provides analgesia for venous cannulation, *Anesthesiology* 72:269, 1990.
Hovorka J, Korttila K: Nitrous oxide does not increase nausea and vomiting following gynaecological laparoscopy, *Can J Anaesth* 36:145, 1989.
Miller K: Analgesia: issues and options, *Emergency* 21:16, 1989.
Thal ER et al: Self-administered analgesia with nitrous oxide: adjunctive aid for emergency medical care systems, *J Am Med Assoc* 242:2418, 1979.
Toulson S: More than a lot of hot air, *Nursing* 4:23, 1990.
Tunstall ME: Implications of pre-mixed gases and apparatus for their administration, *Br J Anaesth* 40:675, 1968.
Wertz EM: Pediatric conscious sedation, *Emergency* 25:19, 1994.

16

Clinical Application of N_2O/O_2 Sedation in Pediatrics

Young children live in a magical world. The thoughts and activities in their world are experienced with an unprejudiced mind and heart. Unfortunately, adults often inadvertently transfer negative attitudes toward dentistry to children. N_2O/O_2 sedation produces a unique euphoria that provides and reinforces a positive attitude toward healthcare in the pediatric patient. Recent evidence suggests that an overwhelming majority of pediatric dentists routinely use N_2O/O_2 sedation in their practices.[1] Thus it can only be surmised that it's great for kids!

I. Child Development

A. Piaget proposed a model for child development that addresses cognitive function or how a child thinks. According to Piaget, children move through four stages of development: sensorimotor, preoperational, concrete operational, and formal operational. He proposed that for cognitive development, the movement from stage to stage was universal and invariant (proceeding in a fixed order)[2] (Table 16-1).
B. These stages give clues about how children should be approached if they are developing normally. Similar to adults, it is common for pediatric patients to have some anxiety regarding medical or dental treatment.
C. There are additional significant factors that affect the development of a child today. Changing patterns of child rearing, parental interactions and attitudes toward professionals, and individual child temperament and personality affect the way a child acts and reacts in any given setting.
D. It is important for health professionals and office staff to be educated about these factors because understanding the pediatric patient's needs and desires and those of the parents is imperative.

II. N_2O-O_2 Use in Pediatrics

A. Pediatric dentistry
   1. The specialty of pediatric dentistry was established in 1948. The reason was simple and quite clear. Children are not small adults in anatomy,

Table 16-1
Piaget's Stages of Child Development

Phase	Language	Fears	Defenses
Sensorimotor Under 18 months	Minimal	Sudden noises New situations Separation from parents	Cry, scream Move away
Preoperational 2-4 years	Developing vocabulary, grammar, language	Not well understood Monsters Dark	Magical Not rational
Preoperational 5-6 years	Language better Simple vocabulary	Can react with shame	Moves away from situation, denial
Operational 7-12 years	Excellent in concrete understanding Abstract less developed	Fears more realistic Fears loss of control Fear of death	Restrained; developing internal defenses
Formal 12-18 years	Full development with language	Mirror adult world Fear of getting hurt Fears of world affairs	Intellectual and rational

physiology, or behavior and they require separate consideration for evaluation, management, and treatment.

2. Wilson[1] reports in a 1993 survey of the membership of the American Academy of Pediatric Dentistry that 89% of the 1758 respondents use N_2O to treat pediatric patients.

a. Of those using N_2O/O_2, the majority of practitioners (87%) used the titration method of administration.

b. The percentage of N_2O administered varied; however, rarely did concentrations exceed 50%.[1]

c. Most respondents indicated that 20% or fewer of their patients required either N_2O/O_2 alone or in combination with other sedatives.[1]

d. Wilson reports that 74% of the respondents do not use any monitors when N_2O/O_2 is used alone. However, when it is used in combination with other sedatives, the pulse oximeter was the single most frequently used monitoring device. A blood pressure cuff and stethoscope were also used when N_2O was combined with other sedatives.[1]

e. When N_2O/O_2 was used alone, only 2% of the respondents had ever experienced a compromised airway. When deeper sedation was achieved using N_2O with other sedatives, the figure affirming experience with a compromised airway rose only to one-third.[1]

f. Primosch et al[3] demonstrated that the delivery of a 40% N_2O/60% O_2 combination significantly improved patient behavior without significantly affecting hemoglobin saturation or type of breath sound.[3]

B. Emergency medicine

1. The use of N_2O in the emergency department has been evaluated for children undergoing procedures such as fracture management, lacera-

tion repair, intravenous cannulation, and other minor surgical procedures.[4-6]

2. Researchers acknowledge the anxiety associated with these procedures
   and the possibility of N_2O to be an effective, noninvasive way to reduce
   anxiety with minimal adverse effects.[4]

3. In cases in which N_2O/O_2 alone was used during fracture reduction, the
   procedure was successful but children reported pain.[7] Hennrikus[7]
   reported greater success when he combined N_2O with a hematoma block
   to provide additional analgesia.

4. During laceration repair, continuous-flow N_2O/O_2 provided pain and
   anxiety relief with minimal adverse effects and shorter recovery than
   when midazolam was used.[8]

C. Gastrointestinal endoscopy

1. The use of N_2O/O_2 for pediatric patients undergoing gastrointestinal
   endoscopy has been evaluated in a pilot study in France.

2. Investigators note the rapid and effective analgesia without heavy sedation in addition to a short recovery period.[9]

3. It is important to keep in mind that using 50% N_2O and 50% O_2 as a
   standard method of administration is contrary to the best and most effective administration technique.

D. Painful procedures

1. N_2O/O_2 has proven beneficial for pediatric patients who must undergo
   repeated painful procedures such as venous cannulation, bone marrow
   aspiration, lumbar punctures, and dressing changes.[10]

2. The most favorable characteristics cited were short recovery time and
   amnestic effects.

III. Pediatric Patient Considerations for Use of N_2O/O_2 Sedation

A. *The attitude of the practitioner and staff is the single most important factor in the
   successful administration of N_2O/O_2 to pediatric patients.*

B. Spontaneous cooperation and willingness of the patient to accept treatment
   is clearly one of the most important factors to consider.

C. Equally as important is whether the patient can and will respond to reason.

D. It must be determined whether the intended treatment can be accomplished
   with N_2O/O_2 sedation or if additional pharmacologic management is
   required.

E. N_2O/O_2 sedation does not require an extensive physical evaluation of the
   child.

1. Anatomic factors that affect the respiratory system such as enlarged tonsils and adenoids are of relative importance because they can cause
   increased resistance to gas movement.

2. In children, middle ear disturbances can become an important factor to
   consider because N_2O can aggravate these conditions.[11]

3. Advise parents to have children avoid eating a heavy meal before the
   appointment.

a. Pediatric patients are far more likely to regurgitate than adults.
b. Aspiration of vomitus is rare but is a very serious and potentially fatal situation.
c. Let patients vomit if they need to vomit. If vomiting occurs, the mouth must be suctioned and the child's airway cleared of vomitus.

F. Weight is usually a most important factor in the administration of proper medication dosages for patients, particularly children. However, weight is not a consideration for N_2O/O_2 administration.

IV. Administration of N_2O/O_2 Sedation to Pediatric Patients

A. The specific technique of administration does not differ from that of the adult. Titration is the single most important concept to follow.

B. The rapid induction technique method of administration has been advocated to gain the attention and cooperation or regain the composure of young children.
1. High concentrations of N_2O (50% or greater) are administered to children, typically ages 3 years and younger.
2. With this technique, crying can be minimized, initially and temporarily. This "settling" phase is short-lived in most cases and allows the child to regain composure.
3. After composure has been attained, the concentration should be reduced.
4. "Crashing" or giving high concentrations of N_2O initially until an injection is given is a technique employed by many pediatric dentists with success in very young children (Figure 16-1).
   a. Remember that N_2O has its own analgesic effects.
   b. This fact should be recognized and used during the injection phase of treatment.

C. Avoid the "roller coaster" effect of sharp increases and decreases in concentrations of N_2O administered.
1. This can make the patient feel nauseous or feel unpleasant about the whole experience.
2. If patients become nauseous, turn down the N_2O and increase the O_2 flow.

D. All child patients should be encouraged to touch, examine, and place the nasal hood on the nose before N_2O administration. Make sure it fits snugly. This can decrease patient anxiety and increase trust in the practitioner.

E. Pulse oximetry is commonly used today and the equipment is relatively inexpensive. A pulse oximeter, although not mandatory for minimal sedation, is recommended for moderate sedation (concentrations of 50% N_2O or greater).

F. Preoperative and postoperative vital sign values are to be recorded.

G. Reservoir bags are available in smaller sizes (e.g., 1 to 2 L) that accommodate tidal volumes of pediatric patients.

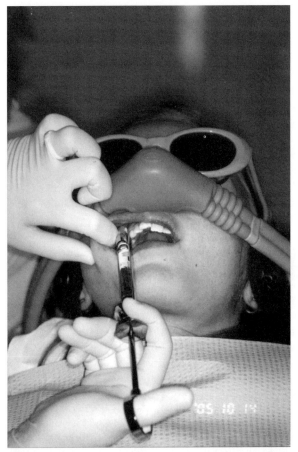

Figure 16-1   Pediatric sedation using N$_2$O/O$_2$. (Courtesy Dr. Elizabeth Barr, Denver, Colorado.)

H. Finally, positive reinforcement (e.g., material or social reward) is usually given for participating rather than how the child participated during a routine visit to a medical or dental office.

V. Safety of Pediatric Patients

A. All patients are important and their safety and welfare is the first priority. However, it is the pediatric patient who captures all of the practitioner's senses of concern and responsibility. An emergency is especially emotionally charged when a child is involved. N$_2$O/O$_2$ provides a measure of safety that practitioners seek when treating pediatric patients.

B. It is not advised to let the child fall asleep under N$_2$O/O$_2$ sedation.
   1. Silent regurgitation is the most engaging concern in this situation.
   2. Maintaining conversation with the child ensures the protective laryngeal and pharyngeal reflexes are intact and the child is able to cough.

3. If a child does fall asleep, a pretracheal scope will alert the practitioner that the airway is not patent.

C. Parents are generally dismissed before the procedure starts if the child is 3 years old or older.

1. Separation breaks the dependent psychologic bond that can worsen a fearful situation. Parents who insist on staying in the operatory are requested to be passive observers.

2. Parents must be informed in detail about the procedure and that the child should be 100% recovered and alert upon discharge.

3. Informed consent must be obtained from the parents for each N_2O/O_2 administration.

D. Concomitant use of other agents with N_2O is a matter of practitioner choice. However, it is important to know the pharmacology of the drugs used and their interaction with each other.

VI. Appointment Length

A. Depending on his/her age, personality, and/or systematic health, a child's attention span is minimal and can rarely be maintained beyond 45 minutes.

B. Do not prolong pediatric appointments. It is important to remember not to prolong appointments with children whether using N_2O/O_2 sedation or not.

REFERENCES

1. Wilson S: A survey of the American Academy of Pediatric Dentistry membership: nitrous oxide and sedation, *Pediatr Dent* 18:287, 1995.
2. Piaget J, Inhelder B: *The psychology of the child*, New York, 1969, Basic Books.
3. Primosch RE et al: Effect of nitrous oxide-oxygen inhalation with scavenging on behavioral and physiological parameters during routine dental treatment, *Pediatr Dent* 21(7):417, 1999.
4. Krauss B: Continuous-flow nitrous oxide: searching for the ideal procedural anxiolytic for toddlers, *Ann Emerg Med* 37(1):61, 2001.
5. Griffin G et al: Nitrous oxide-oxygen sedation for minor surgery: experience in a pediatric setting, *JAMA* 245:2411, 1983.
6. Gamis AS et al: Nitrous oxide analgesia in a pediatric emergency department, *Ann Emerg Med* 18:177, 1989.
7. Hennrikus WL: Self-administered nitrous oxide analgesia for pediatric fracture reductions, *J Pediatr Orthop* 14:538, 1994.
8. Luhmann JD et al: A randomized clinical trial of continuous-flow nitrous oxide and midazolam for sedation of young children during laceration repair, *Ann Emerg Med* 37(1):20, 2001.
9. Michaud L: Nitrous oxide sedation in pediatric patients undergoing gastrointestinal endoscopy, *J Pediatr Gastroenterol Nutr* 28(3):310, 1999.
10. Kanagasundaram SA et al: Efficacy and safety of nitrous oxide in alleviating pain and anxiety during painful procedures, *Arch Dis Child* 84(6):492, 2001.
11. Munson ES: Complications of nitrous oxide anesthesia for ear surgery, *Anes Clin North Am* 11(3):559, 1993.

PART III
ISSUES OF SPECIAL CONSIDERATION

17

Potential Biohazards for Health Personnel Associated with Chronic Exposure to N₂O

N_2O/O_2 sedation has already been discussed as a safe procedure that does not pose health risks for patients. However, chronic exposure for health professionals has been an issue of debate and concern for several years. This chapter provides current and accurate information to clarify this sometimes misunderstood and emotional issue.

I. History of Controversial Literature

A. In 1967, a scientist named Vaisman[1] reported that both male and female anesthesiologists in Russia experienced reproductive problems at a significantly higher rate than the general population. Additionally, Vaisman concluded that these problems were caused by the occupational hazard of being chronically exposed to anesthetic gases. Because N_2O was a common denominator in most all anesthetic applications, it was implicated as the causative agent.

B. In the United States, Cohen et al[2-4] published articles in the 1970s dealing with anesthetic health hazards. One 1980 published study[5] surveyed more than 50,000 dentists and dental assistants who were exposed to trace anesthetics. The results suggested that long-term exposure to anesthetic gases could be associated with an increase in general health problems and reproductive difficulty. In this study, ambient N_2O in the office was not measured and data were collected through memory recall by dental personnel.

C. Since Vaisman's original article the literature has continued to document and describe potential adverse effects of chronic exposure to N_2O. However, this literature has been primarily retrospective; therefore inherent biases in study design were inevitable.[6] Because of these flaws, a definitive relationship between the exposure of an individual to N_2O/O_2 and reproductive sequelae cannot be established. Weinberg, Baird, and Rowland[7] addressed these design flaws and proposed recommendations for future studies of this sort.

D. Also during the 1970s, Bruce, Bach, and Arbit[8] investigated the possibility of N_2O affecting perceptual cognition and psychomotor skills of personnel exposed to varying concentrations of the gas. Their results were widely noted because they reported audiovisual impairment in just hours of exposure to as little as 50 parts per million (ppm). Multiple attempts to reproduce the research results of Bruce, Bach, and Arbit have failed; interestingly, these researchers have retracted their conclusions, indicating the results were not based on biologic factors.[9] The National Institute for Occupational Safety and Health (NIOSH) became interested in these and other results being published and in 1977 evaluated the scavenging potential of the equipment used in both the operating room and the outpatient setting. It was determined that 25 ppm was achievable in the operating room but not attainable in a setting such as a dental operatory. Therefore NIOSH chose 50 ppm to be the maximum exposure limit for personnel in a dental setting.[10] Although this limit has not been strictly enforced by the Occupational Safety and Health Administration (OSHA), it remains the recommended standard to date.

E. Despite the negative publicity N_2O received, other studies in the literature claimed no deleterious health effects associated with chronic exposure to N_2O, especially in low concentrations.[11-13] The controversy continued in the literature and was the subject at professional meetings. Both sides of the issue were published; however, because the effects were questionable, the popularity of N_2O/O_2 sedation waned.

F. It became the work of this author to objectively and scientifically evaluate all the published research to verify the possible relationship of chronic exposure to N_2O and its subsequent effects on human health.

1. In 1995, a worldwide literature search on the topic of biohazards associated with N_2O use was conducted at the University of Colorado. Eight hundred and fifty citations were retrieved, of which 23 met the predetermined criteria for scientific merit.

2. The conclusions drawn from this literature review clearly indicated that there was no scientific basis for the previously established threshold levels for the hospital operating room or the dental setting.

3. This research became the impetus for a meeting of interested parties representing dentistry, government, and manufacturing. A result of the September 1995 meeting, which was sponsored by the ADA's Council on Scientific Affairs and Council on Dental Practice, was the formal position statement that a maximum N_2O exposure limit in parts per million has not been determined.[14] A subsequent report from this meeting indicates that the ADA urges governmental agencies to create new recommendations or regulations dealing with N_2O exposure that are science based.

II. Specific Biologic Issues and Health Concerns

A. Inactivation of methionine synthase is mentioned in Chapters 9 and 18. N_2O interferes with this enzyme, which is linked to vitamin B_{12} metabolism. Vitamin B_{12} is necessary for DNA production and subsequent cellular reproduction.

1. Inactivation of methionine synthase occurs rapidly in rats; exposure to 80% N_2O for only 15 minutes revealed inactivation of the enzyme.[15]

Because of this interference, it was postulated that fetal development may be impaired because of exposure to N_2O. Animal studies using approximately 60% N_2O for 24 hours on pregnant rats produced miscarriage and other fetal abnormalities.[16]

2. Despite flawed research designs, there has been evidence that chronic exposure to high levels of N_2O does have an effect on reproduction.[5] However, to date there is no evidence that a direct causal relationship exists between reproductive health and scavenged low levels of N_2O.[13,15]

3. The deoxyuridine suppression test is a sensitive test used to accurately determine the first signs of biologic effect associated with chronic exposure to N_2O. The test detects the early signs of inactivation of the enzyme methionine synthase. Using this test, Nunn et al[17] found that no alteration of this enzyme occurred in anesthetists exposed to between 150 and 400 ppm.

4. In their research, Sweeney et al[18] showed that the first sign of biologic effect using the deoxyuridine suppression test was at a chronic exposure level of 1800 ppm. Experts in the field concur that the level of 400 ppm, suggested by Sweeney et al, is a reasonable exposure level that is both attainable and significantly below the biologic threshold established by Sweeney et al. The Health and Safety Executive (HSE UK) in the United Kingdom Occupation Exposure Limits set a figure of 100 ppm as a time-weighted average for 8 hours.[19]

5. Because of the significant demands for folic acid during organogenesis (first trimester), postponement of N_2O sedation is recommended. For a pregnant female employed in a setting using N_2O, it is important to know the exposure levels of N_2O and to use all recommended trace gas scavenging methods. Depending on the individual and the situation, that employee should determine whether she should avoid the office setting and any N_2O exposure for the first trimester.

B. Megaloblastic anemia, first described in the 1950s, was found in patients treated with N_2O for tetanus.[20] Leukopenia and reduced megaloblastic erythropoiesis resembling pernicious anemia ensued.

C. Neurologic disorders associated with chronic N_2O exposure appear as myeloneuropathy. Symptoms such as sensory and proprioception impairment may be permanent but are usually temporary with slow recovery.

III. Current Literature

A. Articles published in the 1990s refer primarily to scavenged vs. unscavenged N_2O levels. In the 1990s, practitioners were educated on ways to effectively scavenge trace gas contamination, with the primary method being the evacuation system and the scavenging nasal hood or mask.

1. The scavenging mask system has become standard for all available designs. When expired N_2O is exhaled through the nose, vacuum suction ports transport this gas through the central suction to the outside atmosphere (Figure 17-1). Studies evaluating the scavenging efficacy of masks

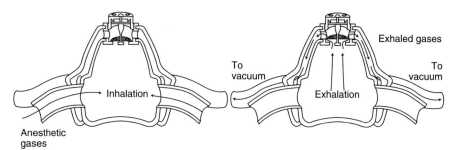

Figure 17-1   Diagram of scavenging nasal hood. (From Malamed SF: *Sedation: a guide to patient management*, St Louis, Mosby, 2003.)

indicate that current models significantly reduce the amount of trace N_2O in the ambient air.[21,22]

2. This evacuation flow rate has been established by NIOSH as optimal at 45 L per minute.

3. Improved mask designs and/or evacuation devices are being investigated as modifications or additions to the current market.[23-27] As technology advances rapidly, no doubt there will be more efficient products. Ongoing research in this area is encouraged.

B. The published literature has served as a vehicle for informing healthcare professionals of the necessity to analyze N_2O exposure levels in their settings and the ways to minimize trace gas. However, there is evidence that some professionals practice without scavenging equipment and without using any other suggested recommendations.[28-30] Using equipment that does not have scavenging capabilities is clearly a breach of the standard of care.

C. A search of the literature since 1995 uncovered many foreign articles referring to the effectiveness of scavenging trace gas. Several note dramatic decreases in parts per million of N_2O in ambient air when using several scavenging methods.[31-38]

IV. Detection and Monitoring of N_2O

A. Infrared (IR) spectrophotometry
1. IR spectrophotometry uses electromagnetic energy to detect levels of N_2O in the atmosphere. This technology can detect levels lower than 1 ppm. Figure 17-2 shows an IR spectrophotometer.

2. Other gases can be detected with this technology as well. An advantage of IR spectrophotometry is the ability to detect minute levels of gas immediately in the ambient air.

3. The instrument can be rented for a reasonable fee and used to instantly detect the presence of N_2O in any setting.

Figure 17-2 Infrared spectrophotometer. (Courtesy Thermo Environmental Instruments, Inc., Franklin, Mass.)

4. This method of analyzing trace gas contamination in the environment is recommended to establish a baseline reference of N_2O exposure levels. Depending on the results, low levels may be confirmed because of the use of scavenging methods; high levels indicate the necessity to implement the recommended scavenging methods. Periodic evaluation with this instrument is advised.
B. Time-weighted average (TWA) dosimetry
   1. It is also possible to determine the amount of N_2O exposure of an individual over time. This method gives an estimate of the amount of exposure to a gas over a specified period.
   2. The badge or vial (similar to a radiation-dosimetry badge) is worn for the recommended period (during exposure or a full workweek) and then returned to the company for analysis. An active material in the badge absorbs the N_2O. The amount is read by an IR spectrophotometer (Figure 17-3) to determine the parts per million of exposure.
   3. An advantage to this system is that it is inexpensive and allows for monitoring in a practice not extensively using N_2O. There are several companies that offer these personal monitoring devices. See Appendix A for reference information.
C. Hand-held monitoring device (Bacharach N_2O Monitor 3010)

Figure 17-3   Time-weighted average dosimetry badge. (Courtesy Assay Technology, Palo Alto, Calif.)

1. A new product to enter the market is a small, lightweight, portable N_2O gas monitor that gives a continuous measure of N_2O in the ambient air (Figure 17-4).
2. The 8-ounce machine that fits in the palm of your hand has both ppm and twa measurement capabilities that are activated with the touch of a button. The internal sampling pump is zeroed with fresh ambient air and measures N_2O in 5 ppm increments up to a 10,000 ppm maximum. The twa capability is available in both real time (over 8 hours) and elapsed time, which begins when the unit is switched on.
3. The monitor can also be used to detect leaks around equipment. Another beneficial feature is its ability to store data for recordkeeping and monitoring purposes.
4. The cost of the unit is not prohibitive and offers a readily available method for assessing occupational risk of exposure to N_2O. See Figure 17-4 and Appendix A for reference information.

V. Scavenging N_2O

A. Scavenging N_2O means minimizing trace amounts of the gas before, during, or after use by the patient.

Figure 17-4   Hand-held N₂O monitoring system. (Courtesy Bacharach, Inc., Pittsburgh, Pa.)

B. The term *scavenging system* traditionally referred to the mask and suction capabilities of the equipment but is currently a term used to identify several methods for the comprehensive removal of trace N₂O.

C. Certain situations are more problematic for scavenging than others.
  1. Patients that are intubated (i.e., tracheal tube) are in a closed-circuit system that affords every opportunity for complete control over trace waste anesthetic gases.
  2. Patients in an ambulatory setting represent a greater opportunity for trace gas loss because of the open circuitry of the sedation machine. N₂O leakage can be found in several places in this setting (Figure 17-5).
  3. Depending on the location of the office (e.g., in a high-rise building), scavenging efforts may be more difficult with regard to ventilation issues.

D. Sources of leakage from the patient
  1. There are several ways that N₂O can leak from the patient. Perhaps the most critical measure to control in this category is patient talking. Whenever patients talk, they are expelling N₂O into the operator's breathing zone. Instruct patients to breathe through their nose and minimize talking.
  2. An ill-fitting mask is a potential source for a significant amount of gas leakage. Ensure a snug, comfortable fit and the appropriate tidal volume before titrating N₂O.

Figure 17-5   Sources of potential N_2O leaks.

3. Other leak sources related to the patient are displacement of the mask during patient movement or restlessness, a technical problem with the mask (e.g., a stuck flutter valve), mouth breathing, or a moustache preventing a tight fit.

E. Sources of leakage other than the patient
   1. Gas can leak at any place of connection on the equipment. This includes the manifold and wall-mounted connections and any hoses associated with each.
   2. Conducting tubing and the reservoir bag are areas of concern. Because of the breakdown of some materials, it is possible for these items to crack and subsequently leak around pleats and/or seams (Figure 17-6).
   3. The soap and water method (Figure 17-7) for determining leaks is recommended for inspecting the areas mentioned in this section. The presence of bubbles after application of the soap and water solution indicates a gas leak.
   4. Door seals and any place where reentry of contaminated air can occur is a potential problem.

F. An evacuation (vacuum) system is used to pull trace gas from the mask into the suction for ultimate dispersal to the outside atmosphere.
   1. Again, the optimal flow rate is 45 L per minute.
   2. Adjustment of this suction rate is critical for effective sedation. Too much suction will make the gas unavailable for the patient, and not enough suction will create trace gas contamination by leakage around the mask.
   3. It is important to periodically check this flow rate during sedation.

Figure 17-6 N_2O leak potential resulting from breakdown of certain materials.

G. Adequate ventilation is an area being investigated for improvement.
   1. In a hospital operating room, fresh-air exchange systems are inherent in the design of the room. In an ambulatory setting such as a dental office there may not be such a provision. Often, air conditioners recirculate ambient air throughout the office, thereby contributing to contamination rather than N_2O elimination. The number of fresh-air exchanges necessary for eliminating trace gas is being investigated.[39]

Figure 17-7   Soap and water solution used to test for N_2O leaks.

2. It is recommended that fresh-air inlets be located in the ceiling and designed to direct the fresh-air supply toward the floor to ensure adequate dilution and mixing of the waste gas. Exhaust register louvers should be located near the floor to allow for adequate flushing of the trace N_2O and to prevent short circuiting of the fresh-air supply.[40]

3. Oscillating room fans can be added to assist in moving the gas to a return vent or to an outside source such as an open window.

4. Monitoring air flow can be accomplished with the use of an electronic micromanometer (Figure 17-8). The AirData Multimeter ADM-850 can detect and measure air velocity, differential pressure measurements, temperature, and air flow. This device is valuable when assessing the adequacy of ventilation in an area. See Figure 17-8 and Appendix A for reference information.

H. Other scavenging strategies

1. Other scavenging devices have been investigated for their ability to assist in minimizing occupational exposure to N_2O and other gases.

2. Local exhaust systems located near the patient's mouth were devised. Noise generated and size of exhaust systems were limitations associated with these devices.[41]

VI. Recommendations and Preventive Measures

A. Monitor the environment for N_2O concentrations.

1. Establish baseline values if equipment is just being installed. For existing equipment, have the ambient air evaluated periodically using an IR spectrophotometer.

2. Monitor the healthcare professional's personal breathing zone (area immediately adjacent to the nose and mouth in a hemisphere forward of the shoulders with a radius of approximately 6 to 9 inches) using twa dosimetry devices.

B. Prevent leakage from the delivery system through proper maintenance and periodic inspection of the equipment.

1. Visually inspect the reservoir bag and conduction tubing for cracks and leaks before each administration.[14]

2. Eliminate or replace loose-fitting connections, loose or deformed slip joints and/or threaded connections, and defective or worn seals or gaskets.

3. Periodically send the sedation equipment back to the manufacturer (depending on their recommendation) for routine evaluation and maintenance. Do not alter, modify, or attempt to adjust this equipment.

C. Control waste N_2O with an appropriate evacuation system that includes securely fitting masks, sufficient evacuation flow rates (45 L/min), and properly vented pumps.

D. Assess the adequacy of room ventilation and air exchange for effectively removing waste N_2O.

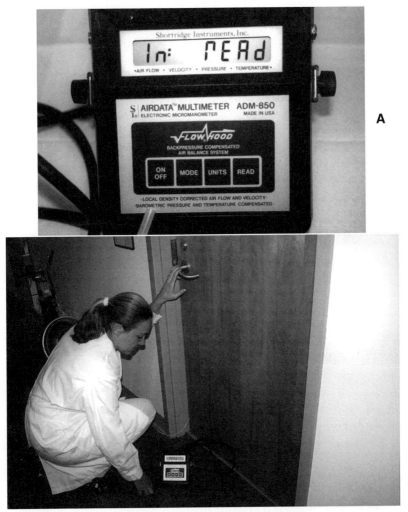

Figure 17-8   Monitoring air flow using an electronic micromanometer.

1. If concentrations are above 25 ppm but less than 150 ppm, it is recommended to increase exhausting capabilities in the area.[42]
2. Supplement local ventilation to capture the N_2O at the source, add oscillating sweep fans, and/or increase the airflow and air exchange to the room.

E. Institute an education program for members of the healthcare team that describes the hazards of N_2O and defines the preventive measures for reducing or eliminating trace gas contamination (Box 17-1).

BOX 17-1
Suggested Office Protocol

1. Possess appropriate delivery system with scavenging capabilities, accurate flowmeter, adequate vacuum, and variety of sizes of masks.
2. Assess the adequacy of ventilation system.
   Vent exhaust to outside.
   Provide fresh air exchange whenever possible.
3. Assess the adequacy of suction system.
   Ensure vacuum at 45 L/min.
   Select appropriate size of mask.
   Establish appropriate tidal volume.
   Discourage patient talking.
4. Assess ambient air for trace gas levels at baseline and periodically thereafter. Periodic personal sampling of personnel should be conducted as well.
5. Assess cylinder attachments, lines, hosing, reservoir bag for leaks. Use IR spectrophotometer and soap and water tests.
6. Calibrate flowmeter(s) every 2 years.

ADA Council on Scientific Affairs.

VII. Summary

A. N_2O/O_2 sedation is a very valuable tool in the ambulatory health setting for the control of pain and anxiety. Practitioners will continue to rely on its effectiveness.
B. To date there is no direct evidence of any causal relationship between chronic low-level exposure to N_2O and potential biologic effects. The maximum safe concentration of N_2O has not been determined; however, every attempt should be made to reduce the level of trace N_2O to exposed health-care personnel. Practitioners cannot be too cautious when their health and that of their co-workers is at stake.
C. Continued research efforts for the scientific advancement of topics related to chronic exposure to N_2O and additional ways to minimize and/or eliminate trace gas contamination are encouraged. Emphasis should be placed on prospective and well-designed studies. Manufacturers should be encouraged to continue their efforts at creating and maintaining effective and efficient equipment.
D. Continuing education should be required of healthcare professionals using N_2O/O_2 sedation, as should evidence of proper training using state-of-the-art equipment and administration techniques.

REFERENCES

1. Vaisman A: Working conditions in surgery and their effect on the health of anesthesiologists, *Eksp Khir Anesteziol* 3:44, 1967.
2. Cohen EN, Belville JW, Brown BW: Anesthesia, pregnancy and miscarriage: a study of operating room nurses and anesthetists, *Anesthesiology* 35:343, 1971.

3. Cohen EN et al: Occupational disease among operating room personnel: a national study, *Anesthesiology* 41:321, 1974.

4. Cohen EN et al: A survey of anesthetic health hazards among dentists: report of an American Society of Anesthesiologists ad hoc committee on the effects of trace anesthetics on the health of operating room personnel, *J Am Dent Assoc* 90:1291, 1975.

5. Cohen EN et al: Occupational disease in dentistry and chronic exposure to trace anesthetic gases, *J Am Dent Assoc* 101:21, 1980.

6. Clark MS, Renehan BW, Jeffers BW: Clinical use and potential biohazards of nitrous oxide/oxygen, *Gen Dent* 45:486, 1997.

7. Weinberg CR, Baird DD, Rowland AS: Pitfalls inherent in retrospective time-to-event studies: the example of time to pregnancy, *Stat Med* 12:867, 1993.

8. Bruce DL, Bach MJ, Arbit J: Trace anesthetic effects on perceptual, cognitive, and motor skills, *Anesthesiology* 40:453, 1974.

9. Yagiela JA: Health hazards and nitrous oxide: a time for reappraisal, *Anesth Prog* 38:1, 1991.

10. Bruce DL, Bach MJ: Trace effects of anesthetic gases on behavioral performance of operating room personnel, HEW publication No (NIOSH) 76-169, Cincinnati, 1976, US Department of Health, Education, and Welfare.

11. Ericson HA, Kallen AB: Hospitalization for miscarriage and delivery outcome among Swedish nurses working in operating rooms in 1973-1978, *Anest Anal* 64:981, 1985.

12. Hemminke K, Kyyronen P, Lindbohm ML: Spontaneous abortions and malformation in the offspring of nurses exposed to anaesthetic gases, cytostatic drugs, and other potential hazards in hospitals based on registered information of outcome, *J Epidemiol Community Health* 39:141, 1985.

13. Rowland AS et al: Reduced fertility among women employed as dental assistants exposed to high levels of nitrous oxide, *New Eng J Med* 327:993, 1992.

14. ADA Council on Scientific Affairs, ADA Council on Dental Practice: Nitrous oxide in the dental office, *J Am Dent Assoc* 128:364, 1997.

15. Eger EI II: Fetal injury and abortion associated with occupational exposure to inhaled anesthetics, *J Am Assoc Nurse Anesth* 59:309, 1991.

16. Fujinagra M, Baden JM, Mazze RI: Susceptible period of nitrous oxide teratogenicity in Sprague-Dawley rats, *Teratology* 40:439, 1989.

17. Nunn JF et al: Serum methionine and hepatic enzyme activity in anaesthetists exposed to nitrous oxide, *Br J Anaesth* 54:593, 1982.

18. Sweeney B et al: Toxicity of bone marrow in dentists exposed to nitrous oxide, *Br Med J* 291:567, 1985.

19. Dookun R et al: Nitrous oxide: past, present, and future, *SAAD Digest* 14(1-2):13, 1997.

20. Lassen JA et al: Treatment of tetanus: severe bone-marrow depression after prolonged nitrous-oxide anaesthesia, *Lancet* 1:527, 1956.

21. Donaldson D, Orr J: A comparison of the effectiveness of nitrous oxide scavenging devices, *J Can Dent Assoc* 55:535, 1989.

22. Certosimo F et al: Clinical evaluation of the efficacy of three nitrous oxide scavenging units during dental treatment, *Gen Dent* p 430, Sept/Oct 2002.

23. Crouch KG, Johnston OE: Nitrous oxide control in the dental operatory: auxiliary exhaust and mask leakage, design, and scavenging flow rate as factors, *Am Ind Hyg Assoc J* 57:272, 1996.

24. Donaldson D, Grabi J: The efficiency of nitrous oxide scavenging devices in dental offices, *J Can Dent Assoc* 55:541, 1989.

25. Ooi R, Joshi P, Soni N: Nitrous oxide/oxygen analgesia: the performance of the MC mask delivery system, *J Royal Soc Med* 85:534, 1992.

26. Shafer SM: Face mask scavenging system, *J Oral Maxillofac Surg* 51:945, 1993.

27. Quarnstrom F: Nitrous oxide safety: how safe is it for staff? What can be done to make it safer? *Dent Today* 18(12):74, 1999.

28. Dunning DG, McFarland K, Safarik M: Nitrous-oxide use. I. Risk of potential exposure and compliance among Nebraska dentists and dental assistants, *Gen Dent* 44:520, 1997.

29. Wilson S: A survey of the American Academy of Pediatric Dentistry membership: nitrous oxide and sedation, *Pediatr Dent* 18:287, 1996.

30. ECRI Reporting System: Hazard update: nitrous oxide cryosurgical units must be scavenged, *Health Devices* 25:306, 1996.

31. Schuyt HC, Verberk MM: Measurement and reduction of nitrous oxide in operating rooms, *Occup Environ Med* 38:1036, 1996.

32. Imberti R, Preseglio I, Imbriani M: Low flow anaesthesia reduces occupational exposure to inhalation anaesthetics, *Acta Anaes Scand* 39:586, 1995.

33. Lucchini R, Toffoletto F, Camerino D: Neurobehavioral functions in operating theatre personnel exposed to anesthetic gases, *Med Lav* 86:27, 1995.

34. Hoerauf KH et al: Occupational exposure to sevoflurane and nitrous oxide in operating room personnel, *Int Arch Occup Environ Health* 69:134, 1997.

35. Chang WP, Kau CW, Hseu SS: Exposure of anesthesiologists to nitrous oxide during pediatric anesthesia, *Ind Health* 35:112, 1997.

36. Ahlborg G Jr, Axelsson G, Bodin L: Shift work, nitrous oxide exposure and subfertility among Swedish midwives, *Int J Epidemiol* 25:783, 1996.

37. Breum NO, Kann T: Elimination of waste anaesthetic gases from operating theatres, *Acta Anaesthesiol Scand* 32:388, 1988.

38. Hobbhahn J et al: Occupational exposure to sevoflurane, halothane and nitrous oxide during paediatric anaesthesia, *Anaesthesia* 52:215, 1997.

39. Borganelli GN, Primosch RE, Henry RJ: Operatory ventilation and scavenger evacuation rate influence on ambient nitrous oxide levels, *J Dent Res* 72:1275, 1993.

40. Howard WR: Nitrous oxide in the dental environment: assessing the risk, reducing the exposure, *J Am Dent Assoc* 128:356, 1997.

41. Byhahn C et al: Surgeon's occupational exposure to nitrous oxide and sevoflurane during pediatric surgery, *World J Surg* 25(9):1109, 2001.

42. McGlothlin JD, Crouch KG, Mickelsen RL: Control of nitrous oxide in dental operatories, DHHS No (NIOSH) 94-129, Cincinnati, 1994, US Department of Health and Human Services, Public Health Service, Centers for Disease Control and Prevention, National Institute for Occupational Safety and Health, Division of Physical Sciences and Engineering, Engineering Control Technology Branch.

18

N$_2$O Abuse Issues

N$_2$O has been used for recreational purposes since its discovery in the late eighteenth century. Sir Humphrey Davy and Dr. Gardner Colton traveled the world proclaiming the exhilarating effects of inhaling N$_2$O in those early days. Inhaling the gas was popular at social gatherings during that time and is still done at parties today. N$_2$O abuse is an issue about which healthcare professionals should be aware. When chronically abused, N$_2$O can have serious health ramifications. N$_2$O should be given the same respect that is given to all drugs.

I. Inhalant Abuse

A. All drugs that produce euphoria have the potential to be abused, whether they are injected, swallowed, or inhaled. However, not all drugs that can be abused through inhalation are defined as "inhalants." The term *inhalant* applies to a group of substances that produce psychoactive reactions and are defined solely by their route of administration.[1] The commonality between these substances is that they are volatile and used to alter consciousness. Typical modes of administration are nasal inhalation called *sniffing* or *snorting*, inhaling contents from a bag or *bagging*, holding a saturated rag in the mouth and inhaling or *huffing*, and spraying the substance directly into the mouth.[1]

B. Inhalants are generalized to three categories: volatile solvents, nitrites, and N$_2$O.[2] Solvents are abused much more than nitrites and N$_2$O.

C. Inhaling chemicals found in a variety of household products is a method of achieving a quick, exhilarating high. It is particularly unfortunate that this type of inhalant abuse appears to be most common among children and adolescents. Inhalants were second behind marijuana as the most commonly used illicit drugs by teenagers in the 1990s.[3] Studies in the 1980s indicated that 18.6% of U.S. high school seniors had practiced inhaling chemicals at least once; specific states claimed even higher incidence figures and younger users.[4] A 1993 report from the National Institute on Drug Abuse[5] (NIDA) indicates approximately 17% of U.S. adolescents say they have sniffed inhalants. For youth and others who may be disadvantaged financially, inhalants present a way of "getting high" that is cheap and easily obtained.[4]

D. These younger users claim a variety of favorite inhalant products. Euphoria-producing chemicals, found in commonly used products, are readily available.

    1. Examples of volatile solvents that are inhaled include fuels such as gasoline, butane, and propane; solvents; paint and paint thinner; rubber cement; airplane glue; hair spray; shoe polish; nail polish remover; deodorants; lubricating cooking sprays; insect repellent; and typewriter correction fluid (Box 18-1).

    2. Typewriter correction fluid is one of the favored inhalants. It contains the chemical 1,1,1-trichloroethane or trichloroethylene. Through 1988, abuse of this substance was responsible for 27 reported fatalities. A leading manufacturer incorporated mustard oil into its product to discourage abuse.[4] Health risks from inhaling this product include liver damage, cranial neuropathy, and cardiac toxicity.[4]

E. Many inhalants are CNS depressants that produce sensations similar to the effects of sedation and anesthesia. However, abusers are looking for the exhilarating, euphoric, visually stimulating effects. Effects are produced in less than 1 minute and are usually not long lasting. Some experienced users claim to feel effects for up to 45 minutes and can therefore time their experiences to prolong their exuberance for hours.[4] Disorientation can occur; nausea and vomiting have been reported, as well as sneezing, coughing, and salivation.[6]

F. Obviously these products are sold legally and are relatively inexpensive. They are found at home and in the garage. They are purchased in grocery, hardware, and drug stores. They can be packaged in small containers that are easily hidden. Most often, purchase of such products causes no suspicion. However, in some areas local sale restrictions may apply.

G. Other risk groups for abuse of these inhalants include those who may be occupationally exposed to the products. Those at risk may be janitors, painters, dry cleaning personnel, automobile repair workers, or hairstylists.[4]

H. Amyl nitrite and butyl nitrite ("poppers") are muscle relaxants inhaled primarily to intensify and prolong sexual experiences. Marketed as room deodorizers these products may produce symptoms such as headaches, blurred vision, and cardiac arrhythmia.[4]

BOX 18-1
Commonly Inhaled Substances

Typewriter correction fluid
Butane, gasoline, propane
Paint and paint thinner
Rubber cement, model glue
Hair spray, cooking spray, deodorant spray
Insect repellants
N_2O

I. N$_2$O falls into the inhalant classification as well. It has similar pharmacokinetic properties to those products listed above. It is relatively inexpensive, readily accessible, legal to purchase, and produces a rapid, euphoric high. Users recommend its use to others claiming that it produces feelings of floating or flying; vivid, visual, colorful images; and loss of all inhibitions, making the user feel invincible. Of course the negative side effects like fatigue, fainting, nausea, and cardiac arrest are rarely mentioned.

J. Death has been associated with inhalant abuse. Death can occur the first time a person inhales a toxic substance. Cardiac dysfunction, respiratory depression, and asphyxiation are the likely causes of death.[7] Suicidal and accidental deaths have also been associated with inhalant abuse. Bowen et al[8] report 52 deaths in Virginia between 1987 and 1996 that were associated with inhalation compounds. Thirty-nine of the deaths resulted from acute voluntary exposure.[8] Victims' ages ranged from 13 to 42 years with 19 years being the average age when death occurred.

II. N$_2$O Abuse

A. N$_2$O users tend to be somewhat older than those inhaling solvents and fuels, etc. As when it was first introduced, N$_2$O is popular today at college social activities such as parties and concerts and may be advertised in college papers or flyers. N$_2$O etiquette can be found in high-society magazines; reference to its use at elite parties can be found in novels. Now instructions for its use can be found even on the Internet.

B. Health professionals who have ready access to the gas are noted recreational users. In general, health professionals have access to many drugs, and abuse is often not limited to one drug. Anesthesiologists and those in training, students in psychiatric and maxillofacial programs, physicians, and dentists are groups cited in the literature as being substance abusers.[9,10] In a 1977 anonymous survey of medical and dental students, 20% admitted to using N$_2$O socially.[11]

C. N$_2$O is easy to obtain for recreational use and is found in several forms.
 1. Because it is commonly found compressed in cylinders and used for medical and dental purposes, it is easy to locate in hospitals, clinics, dental offices, etc.
  a. Several agencies have reported stolen cylinders from such places. Individuals employed in such a setting may be able to use the gas on site rather than take the risk of stealing the cylinder.
  b. Distribution centers where cylinders of N$_2$O are filled and distributed to various sites report occasional robbery attempts. Large cylinders previously stored outside of buildings have been moved indoors for security.
 2. N$_2$O is also used in the auto racing industry; it supports combustion and is used as an engine-boosting agent. However, N$_2$O used for this purpose is often mixed with sulfur dioxide. Inhaling this noxious mixture is likely to render a person ill with vomiting, headache, and diarrhea.

Figure 18-1   Whipping cream charger "whippet."

3. Messina and Wynne,[12] researching homemade N_2O, produced the gas according to instructions widely distributed in "head shops" and claim that the process was easy and inexpensive. They also report that significant concentrations of nitrogen dioxide and nitric oxide are produced with this method. These substances are toxic and can cause transient pulmonary toxicity and tissue damage.

4. N_2O is approved by the Food and Drug Administration (FDA) as a food ingredient because the dairy industry uses it as a whipping cream propellant. The gas expands into the cream causing it to whip into foam. When used for these legitimate purposes, N_2O is found in 3-inch-long containers called *whippets* (Figure 18-1). These containers hold approximately 4 to 5 L of N_2O. These products are also misused for recreational purposes.

   a. In addition to the whippet charger, a "cracker" and a balloon must be purchased (Figure 18-2). A balloon is attached to one end while the

Figure 18-2   Whippet assembly for recreational misuse.

charger is placed between the two halves of the cracker. A pointed extension inside the cracker pierces the diaphragm on the charger as the two halves are screwed together. The gas is expelled out of the charger and fills the balloon.

5. Similarly, approximately 3 L of N$_2$O is found in aerosol cans of whipping cream. It is the N$_2$O that whips the cream coming out of the can. Figure 18-3 illustrates N$_2$O listed as a propellant.

   a. This activity becomes a game as users try to "hit" off of a can in a grocery store without buying the product. This "grocery store high" was reported in the psychiatric literature in 1978.[13] Restaurants have reported the necessity of locking the supply of whipping cream cans to prevent restaurant servers from sampling the N$_2$O while on the job.

   b. To prohibit inhaling N$_2$O from the aerosol can without purchasing it, manufacturers have considered wrapping the entire can in tamper-resistant plastic.

   c. N$_2$O can also be found in chargers that are similar in size to a seltzer bottle. Again, the legitimate use is for creating whipped cream; however, those misusing it inhale the contents directly from the bottle or dispel it into balloons.[14]

D. Because of the pharmacokinetics of the drug, N$_2$O is rarely detected in routine urine tests.[15] Therefore users may substitute N$_2$O for other more detectable drugs, especially when driving. However, there have been reports of youth involved in fatal car accidents when under the influence of N$_2$O.[14]

Figure 18-3   Aerosol whipping cream can ingredient list; note the propellant listed is N$_2$O.

III. Health Hazards Associated with Chronic Exposure to N$_2$O

A. N$_2$O has been shown to affect vitamin B$_{12}$ metabolism. It oxidizes the cobalt ion in the vitamin B$_{12}$ cofactor, rendering the enzyme methionine synthase inactive in folate metabolic pathways. Methionine synthase plays a vital role in the production of DNA. Megaloblastic hematopoiesis and leukopenia result after prolonged exposure to N$_2$O.[16]

1. For most healthy surgical or ambulatory patients undergoing N$_2$O/O$_2$ sedation, the effects of inactivated methionine synthase are temporary and insignificant. There appears to be a greater risk for pregnant women, those with impaired wound healing capabilities, and for those with existing vitamin B$_{12}$ deficiencies.[16]

2. Studies on laboratory animals have shown that enzyme inactivation occurs rapidly during N$_2$O overexposure and that recovery is slow.[16,17] Animal studies have also shown evidence of fetal toxicity resulting in skeletal abnormalities and miscarriages after significant exposure to N$_2$O in terms of concentration and time.[16]

3. Several studies with humans revealed significant hematopoietic changes as well; the earliest report was cited in 1956.[18-20] Research has confirmed this consequence over the years. An excellent reference list to this subject can be found in Eger's text,[21] *Nitrous Oxide, N$_2$O.*

4. Individuals who are chronically exposed to N$_2$O through its recreational use or occupational use in unscavenged areas may be at risk for hematopoietic changes and other sequelae. Chapter 17 provides further details on the biohazard and scavenging issues associated with trace gas contamination.

5. Those persons who are vitamin B$_{12}$ deficient may not be aware of the deficiency until the N$_2$O exposure produces neurologic changes.[22,23]

   a. Practitioners reveal in the literature instances in which patients with preexisting vitamin B$_{12}$ deficiencies, folate abnormalities or inherited folate disorders, or those taking antifolate medication may be at risk for adverse effects when exposed to N$_2$O.[24] A reported case of subacute combined degeneration of the spinal cord occurred postoperatively after surgery using N$_2$O in a patient found to be vitamin B$_{12}$ deficient.[25]

   b. It has been suggested that a vitamin B$_{12}$ supplement be taken by women exposed to N$_2$O as a method for reducing fetotoxic effects.[22] The possibility of biochemical protection exists for other compromised individuals as well. It has been suggested that preoperative concentration levels of vitamin B$_{12}$ be established and deficiencies corrected to avoid possible neurologic complications.[26]

   c. Researchers agree that this is an area in need of continued study.

B. Neurologic side effects have been associated with chronic use of N$_2$O. Several reports in the literature cite peripheral neuropathy in individuals who indicate habitual use of N$_2$O.[27]

1. Neurologic symptoms have been reported primarily by individuals who have admitted using N$_2$O recreationally; however, in some cases, affected individuals were exposed to significant amounts of unscavenged N$_2$O in hospitals or during dental surgery.[28] Symptoms relating to peripheral neuropathy are evidenced by tingling and numbness in the extremities, weakness and incoordination, lack of strength and dexterity in the hands, slowed gait, and positive Lhermitte's sign (electric shock feeling upon flexion of the neck).[29-31]

2. Often the neuropathic symptoms are not immediate; they may appear several months into the overexposure period.[28] Generally, neurologic function slowly returns to normal after termination of overexposure to the gas. This return is gradual and in some cases may not be complete.[28]

3. The cases of overexposure reported in the literature are primarily dentists or other health professionals who deliver N$_2$O to patients without proper scavenging equipment.[32] Other cases are young adults recreationally inhaling N$_2$O from whipping cream chargers.[29,32] Most of the overexposure incidents reported were periods of 1 to 2 hours per day, at least three times a week, and for periods of several months to years.[27,32] In some cases individuals reported falling asleep and incurring up to 4 hours of exposure; one individual admitted self-administration of 2 to 4 hours per day and another admitted 6 to 7 hours per day.[32]

C. Frostbite has been cited as a consequence of exposure to N$_2$O. An adult male experienced an accident at his place of employment in which a pressure-reducing valve broke from an N$_2$O cylinder exposing the man to the gas. He was treated for life-threatening pharyngeal swelling from severe frostbite of the oral cavity.[33] More significant are reports of individuals sniffing N$_2$O straight from the cylinder, causing their mouths, lips, and cheeks to freeze to the extent that tissue necrosed to a fourth-degree burn.[34] The temperature of the N$_2$O gas streaming from a cylinder may be as low as −55° C.[33] In one instance, an individual became so disoriented from inhaling the gas that he was unaware that his cheek was in contact with the gas and cylinder for a prolonged period.[34]

D. There have been reports of pneumothorax or pneumomediastinum resulting from the pressure released from a whippet charger. In one instance, actual rupture of alveolar walls occurred, causing interstitial emphysema.[35]

E. Several reports of asphyxial death from N$_2$O are stated in the literature.[36-39] All victims were using N$_2$O recreationally. Several victims have been health-care workers, others worked in restaurants, and some were users outside of the workplace.

1. The reported deaths of healthcare workers usually involve cylinder apparatus with face masks. Details surrounding the instances reveal victims being found near tanks in healthcare settings.

2. Other reports describe victims being discovered with plastic bags over their heads and belts or similar devices around their necks to keep the bags closed. In these situations chargers are frequently used and are discharged inside the plastic bag.

a. Wagner et al[15] recreated the scenario of discharging a whipping cream charger inside a plastic bag. Within 10 seconds of discharging, the 21% O_2 concentration found in ambient air inside the bag had dropped to 13% and the N_2O concentration escalated to 59%. Within 1 minute the O_2 concentration had fallen to 10%.

b. Unconsciousness occurs either from the hypoxia or the drug concentration, and death results when available O_2 is depleted to a level that does not support life.[15] Death by this means sometimes may be sought intentionally and other times may be accidental.

3. In one case, N_2O was implicated as the cause for an autoerotic asphyxial death. The victim had created a method of delivering N_2O through an outdated and modified anesthesia machine, and sexual material describing bondage and other autoerotic methods was found at the scene.[40]

IV. Sexual Phenomena Associated with N_2O

A. Euphoric effects have been associated with N_2O since it was first introduced. Some reports in the literature have indicated that hallucinations, visualizations, and auditory illusions have resulted from N_2O abuse.[41] There have also been situations in which aberrations of a sexual nature have been reported.[42]

1. Allegations of sexual impropriety have been made against health professionals after patients were sedated with N_2O/O_2. These complaints were taken to court for prosecution, but in the majority of cases the charges were dismissed. However, continued licensure was subject to the discretion of the state's licensing board.

2. Specific cases reported have been primarily against male practitioners by female patients. The cases report claims such as the patient falling asleep and being frightened by a vision, pressure sensations in the genital region, becoming sexually stimulated, feeling naked, dreaming, and fantasizing.[42]

3. Jastak and Malamed[42] report that in all of those instances, concentrations of N_2O higher than 50% were used. They also indicate that no other personnel accompanied the dentist during the sedation experience.[42] They recommend that a third party be present at all times and that N_2O concentrations greater than 50% be avoided.

4. Lambert[43] suggests that hypnosis is potentiated by N_2O. He suggests that a person may experience a hypnotic state spontaneously or by the suggestive language of the professional while N_2O is being administered. Lambert[43] recommends that practitioners regard their statements in a professional manner without lending comments that could be misinterpreted. He recommends suggesting visual imagery such as a beach scene to avoid the patient's own imaging.

B. Obviously the allegation of sexual impropriety can create uncomfortable situations. Use common sense when using N_2O; do not place yourself in potentially incriminating situations. Practice with a third party in the vicinity who is educated on the effects of N$_2$O. Titrate to the appropriate end-point of sedation to avoid high concentrations of N$_2$O and oversedation symptoms.

V. Addictive Nature of N$_2$O

A. Compared with other drugs, N$_2$O abuse is low.[14] It is not listed among the most commonly abused drugs. This drug has been used for 150 years without mention of significant abuse and addiction problems.
B. Evidence exists that suggests N$_2$O is involved with the endogenous opioid system directly at a receptor site and/or indirectly by activating opioid neurotransmitters.
   1. Also indicated is the fact that N$_2$O may be considered a partial opioid agonist, making it less addictive than a full agonist such as morphine.[44]
   2. Autotolerance may be an issue with N$_2$O, indicating that the body rapidly becomes tolerant to its effects.[15]
C. Compared with other drugs, N$_2$O abuse does not exist as a public health concern. Alcohol, nicotine, and cannabis have been cited as the most commonly used nonmedical drugs.[45] However, it is still important to be aware of its recreational use among youth and health professionals in particular.

VI. Legislation and Regulation Issues

A. Currently there are few regulations governing the sale or purchase of N$_2$O. Distributors are ethically obligated to confirm that their customers are purchasing the drug for appropriate use; however, there are no control measures to ensure that this is happening. Those selling N$_2$O for purposes other than appropriate use may be held responsible for their actions. In March 2001, "delivering a misbranded drug into interstate commerce" was the charge that led an Arizona man to 15 months in prison and a fine of $40,000. His sale of N$_2$O in whipped cream chargers led to the death of a college student.[46]
B. Warning labels can be found on cylinders, whippets, and whipping cream containers containing N$_2$O. The labels recommend that users be familiar with the administration and properties of the drug and that misuse could be harmful.
C. The Compressed Gas Association Foundation, the CGA, and the NWSA have been active in informing the public about the concern of N$_2$O misuse. The Nitrous Oxide Abuse Task Force was established in 1994 by the CGA and NWSA. They created the Sales and Security Guidelines for the Safe Use/Handling of Nitrous Oxide.[47] The guidelines provide suggestions and information to producers, repackagers, distributors, carriers, and legitimate users of the gas. See Appendix A for references to this information. Fifty-nine associations were targeted by the task force to receive these guidelines. They

range from healthcare and restaurants to auto racing, law enforcement, and trucking.

D. In addition to these guidelines, the CGA and NWSA are working with other organizations to tighten distribution policies and develop strong codes of ethics for voluntary implementation. They also provide assistance to those working with law enforcement individuals dealing with N$_2$O misuse issues.

E. Legislatively, these organizations have been instrumental in assisting the development of model state legislation that would discourage illicit N$_2$O use by prohibiting unlawful possession and/or distribution. Violations are punishable by law. Several states have been on the forefront of this issue and have already been successful in enacting legal regulations. States to be commended for their involvement in this subject are Maryland, West Virginia, Illinois, California, Georgia, and Florida. The recent law in Florida makes it illegal for any person to possess, distribute, or sell N$_2$O. In addition, the law could require violators to participate in a substance abuse program.[48]

REFERENCES

1. Brouette T, Anton R: Clinical review of inhalants, *Am J Addictions* 10:79, 2001.
2. Weir E: Inhalant use and addiction in Canada, *CMAJ* 164(3):397, 2001.
3. Edwards RW, Oetting ER: Inhalant use in the United States, *Natl Inst Drug Abuse Res Monogr Ser* 148:8, 1995.
4. Schwartz RJ: When to suspect inhalant abuse, *Patient Care* 30:39, 1989.
5. National Institute on Drug Abuse Website: www.nida.nih.gov.
6. McHugh MJ: The abuse of volatile substances, *Ped Clin North Am* 34:333, 1987.
7. Adgey AA, Johnston PW, McMechan S: Sudden cardiac death and substance abuse, *Resuscitation* 29(3):219, 1995.
8. Bowen SE et al: Deaths associated with inhalant abuse in Virginia from 1987 to 1996, *Drug Alcohol Depend* 53:239, 1999.
9. Gillman MA: Nitrous oxide abuse in perspective, *Clin Neuropharmacol* 15:297, 1992.
10. From RP: Substance dependence and abuse by anesthesia care providers. In Rogers M et al, editors: *Principles and practice of anesthesiology*, St Louis, 1993, Mosby.
11. Rosenberg H, Orkin FK, Springstead J: Abuse of nitrous oxide, *Anesth Analg* 58:104, 1979.
12. Messina FV, Wynne JW: Homemade nitrous oxide: no laughing matter, *Ann Intern Med* 96:333, 1982.
13. Block SH: The grocery store high, *Am J Psychiatry* 135:126, 1978.
14. Murray MJ, Murray WJ: Nitrous oxide availability, *J Clin Pharm* 20:202, 1980.
15. Wagner SA et al: Asphyxial deaths from the recreational use of nitrous oxide, *J Forensic Sci* 37:1008, 1992.
16. Nunn JF, Chanarin I: Nitrous oxide inactivates methionine synthetase. In Eger EI II: *Nitrous oxide N$_2$O*, New York, 1985, Elsevier Science Publishing.
17. Londo H, Osborne ML: Nitrous oxide has multiple deleterious effects on cobalamin metabolism and causes decreases in activities of mammalian cobalamin dependent enzymes, *J Clin Invest* 67:1270, 1981.
18. Lassen JC et al: Treatment of tetanus: severe bone marrow depression after prolonged nitrous-oxide anaesthesia, *Lancet* 1:527, 1956.
19. Amess JA et al: Megaloblastic haemopoiesis in patients receiving nitrous oxide, *Lancet* 2:339, 1978.

20. Skacel PO et al: Studies on the haemopoietic toxicity of nitrous oxide in man, *Br J Haematol* 53:189, 1983.
21. Eger EI II: *Nitrous oxide, N$_2$O,* New York, 1985, Elsevier Science Publishing.
22. Ostreicher JS: Vitamin B$_{12}$ supplements as protection against nitrous oxide inhalation, *New York State Dent J* 60:47, 1994.
23. Butzkueven H, King JO: Nitrous oxide myelopathy in an abuser of whipped cream bulbs, *J Clin Neurosci* 7(1):73, 2000.
24. Wyatt SS, Gill RS: An absolute contraindication to nitrous oxide, *Anaesthesia* 54(3):307, 1999.
25. Beltramello A et al: Subacute combined degeneration of the spinal cord, *J Neurol Neurosurg Psychiatry* 64(4):563, 1998.
26. Mayall M: Vitamin B$_{12}$ deficiency and nitrous oxide, *Lancet* 352(9163):1529, 1999.
27. Kunkel DB: The toxic emergency, *Emerg Med* 19:79, 1987.
28. Layzer RB: Myeloneuropathy after prolonged exposure to nitrous oxide, *Lancet* 2:1227, 1978.
29. Sahenk Z et al: Polyneuropathy from inhalation of N$_2$O cartridges through a whipped-cream dispenser, *Neurology* 28:485, 1978.
30. Layzer RB, Fishman RA, Schafer JA: Neuropathy following abuse of nitrous oxide, *Neurology* 28:504, 1978.
31. Paulson GW: "Recreational" misuse of nitrous oxide, *J Am Dent Assoc* 98:410, 1979.
32. Gutmann L, Johnsen D: Nitrous oxide-induced myeloneuropathy: report of cases, *J Am Dent Assoc* 103:239, 1981.
33. Svartling N et al: Life-threatening airway obstruction from nitrous oxide induced frostbite of the oral cavity, *Anaesth Intensive Care* 24(6):717, 1996.
34. Hwang JC, Himel HN, Edlich RF: Frostbite of the face after recreational misuse of nitrous oxide, *Burns* 22:152, 1996.
35. LiPuma JP, Wellman J, Stern HP: Nitrous oxide abuse: a new cause for pneumomediastinum, *Radiology* 145:602, 1982.
36. Suruda AJ, McGlothlin JD: Fatal abuse of nitrous oxide in the workplace, *J Occup Med* 32:682, 1990.
37. Garriott J, Petty CS: Death from inhalant abuse: toxicological and pathological evaluation of 34 cases, *Clin Toxicology* 16:305, 1980.
38. Chadly A, Marc B, Barres D: Suicide by nitrous oxide poisoning, *Am J For Med Path* 10:330, 1989.
39. Winek CL, Wahba WW, Rozin L: Accidental death by nitrous oxide inhalation, *Forensic Sci Int* 73:139, 1995.
40. Leadbeatter S: Dental anesthetic death: an unusual autoerotic episode, *Am J For Med Path* 9:60, 1988.
41. Steinberg H: Abnormal behavior induced by nitrous oxide, *Br J Psychol* 47:183, 1956.
42. Jastak JT, Malamed SF: Nitrous oxide sedation and sexual phenomena, *J Am Dent Assoc* 101:38, 1980.
43. Lambert C: Sexual phenomena hypnosis and nitrous oxide sedation, *J Am Dent Assoc* 101:990, 1982.
44. Gillman MA: Nitrous oxide, an opioid addictive agent, *Am J Med* 81:97, 1986.
45. Kreek MJ: Multiple drug abuse patterns and medical consequences. In Meltzer HY, editor: *Psychopharmacology: the third generation of progress,* New York, 1987, Raven Press.
46. Meadows M: Arizona man sentenced for selling nitrous oxide, *FDA Consumer* p 33, May-June 2001.

47. Compressed Gas Association Code-201: *Nitrous oxide sales and security recommended guidelines*, Arlington, Va, 1995, Compressed Gas Association.
48. Tuck MG: Law ups ante on nitrous oxide possession and distribution, *J Dent Technol* 17(7):34, 2000.

SUGGESTED READINGS

Dohrn CS et al: Reinforcing effects of extended inhalation of nitrous oxide in humans, *Drug Alcohol Depend* 31:265, 1993.
Dzoljic M et al: Behavioral and electrophysiological aspects of nitrous oxide dependence, *Brain Res Bull* 33:25, 1994.
Pollard TG: Relative addiction potential of major centrally-active drugs and drug classes—inhalants and anesthetics, *Adv Alcohol Subst Abuse* 9:149, 1990.

19
Ethical and Legal Considerations Regarding N₂O Administration

Healthcare professionals are ethically and legally responsible for providing the best care that is possible for each patient. Practitioners are also required to abide by the laws and rules governing their discipline in their area (e.g., state, province, or country). It is vitally important to be educated on all aspects of N_2O/O_2 sedation and be legally certified or licensed by a governing agency when necessary. And, as stated numerous times in this text, it is imperative to follow the ASA Practice Guidelines for Sedation and Analgesia by Nonanesthesiologists because these will be the standards to which your actions will be compared should legal and/or ethical concerns be expressed.

I. Legal Requirements Associated with N_2O/O_2 Administration

A. Depending on the discipline and the governing body regulating the requirements of practice within the discipline, there are rules to abide by regarding the administration of N_2O/O_2 sedation.
   1. There are widespread variations among disciplines as to who may administer and/or monitor the N_2O/O_2 sedation procedure; the profession may determine who is or is not eligible to provide this type of service and under what conditions it may be administered. These parameters of practice are monitored by the appropriate governing agency, whose purpose is to protect the public.
      a. Depending on the discipline, a practitioner may only be legally allowed to monitor a patient under N_2O/O_2 sedation and not be allowed to administer the drug. This prohibits the individual from titrating N_2O to the patient. This may be the case for certain levels of auxiliaries within a discipline (Boxes 19-1 and 19-2).
   2. In addition, the law outlines the level of supervision necessary for this procedure. In dentistry, states that allow auxiliaries such as dental hygienists to administer N_2O require that the procedure be under the direct supervision of a dentist.
B. Because there are so many legal variations of rules that are discipline specific, it is critical to be informed of the codified law and administrative rules applicable within each state and then practice only within the scope of that law.

BOX 19-1
States That Allow Dental Hygienists to Administer and Monitor N₂O/O₂ Sedation
(as of November 2002)

Alaska
Arizona
Arkansas
California
Colorado
Idaho
Illinois
Iowa
Kansas
Kentucky
Minnesota
Mississippi
Nevada
New York
Oklahoma
Oregon
South Dakota
Tennessee
Utah
Washington

C. It is also legally mandated that informed consent be obtained from the patient or parent or guardian before the administration of N_2O/O_2 sedation. It is prudent practice to confirm the acquisition of informed consent with a patient's or parent's signature at each visit.

II. Appropriate Education for N₂O/O₂ Administration

A. Governing boards and licensing agencies may require a specified course of training in the area of N_2O/O_2 sedation before practitioners can incorporate this procedure into their clinical practices.
  1. Often, proof of successful completion of an approved course on the subject is required. Approved courses usually consist of both didactic and clinical components, totaling a specified minimum number of hours.
  2. After successful completion of such a course of study and probable fee payment, the practitioner may be granted a permit or license to administer N_2O/O_2 sedation.
  3. Most often, students completing their professional curriculum are exempt from additional coursework in this area unless this information was not part of the professional program. In such a case the student is subject to the same requirements as those without the necessary education.
B. It may be favorable for a previously educated practitioner to participate in an N_2O/O_2 sedation refresher course. Updated material, new equipment, or a review of the appropriate administration technique may be presented,

---

BOX 19-2
States That Allow Dental Assistants to Monitor N$_2$O/O$_2$ Sedation
(as of November 2002)

Alabama
Arizona
Arkansas
California
Colorado
Florida
Georgia
Hawaii
Idaho
Iowa
Kentucky
Minnesota
Mississippi
Missouri
Montana
Nebraska
New Mexico
North Carolina
North Dakota
Oklahoma
Oregon
South Dakota
Tennessee
Texas
Washington

---

which could enhance the success of this procedure in clinical practice. We have found that those practitioners participating in review courses return to their practices with a renewed appreciation for the drug and its potential. They value the reinforcement of how the procedure is making their practice successful while providing a valuable service to their patients.

III. Ethical Responsibilities

A. In addition to legal practice guidelines for administering N$_2$O/O$_2$ sedation, there are ethical aspects to consider. N$_2$O/O$_2$ sedation is available for reducing a patient's pain and anxiety before performing a clinical procedure. It is unethical for a healthcare professional to knowingly administer N$_2$O to a patient for any other reason (e.g., thrill seeking).
B. The abuse potential of N$_2$O has been discussed (see Chapter 18). It is the responsibility of the practitioner to ensure that tanks are properly stored and locked securely so that the likelihood of others stealing a tank or abusing N$_2$O is minimized.
C. Do not abuse N$_2$O yourself. There are significant health risks and complications that could affect you permanently. Seek help if necessary. Also, assist others if you suspect or recognize that they may have a problem.

D. Administer N_2O/O_2 using the recommended titration technique. Use updated, state-of-the-art equipment provided by the manufacturers because the delivery systems currently available undergo stringent quality control and safety measures.[1] Use recommended scavenging techniques and procedures for minimizing trace gas contamination to exposed personnel (see Chapter 17).

IV. Prudent Practice Guidelines

A. Avoid allegations of sexual misconduct. The propensity exists for a patient to become sexually stimulated or dream or hallucinate sexual situations while sedated with N_2O. There are obvious ways to avoid allegations of sexual misconduct. Common sense is all that is necessary in most cases.

1. Use the appropriate technique and titrate to the exact level of appropriate sedation. Most patients achieve this endpoint at N_2O concentrations less than 50%. If the patient requires a percentage higher than 50%, the operator should be alerted to the fact that cumulative effects of the drug may quickly change the level of sedation and that this range is considered high risk for dreaming or fantasizing.

2. Always have a third party in the room during the procedure as a witness against false accusations.[1]

3. Do not place yourself in a potentially incriminating situation, such as an after-hours appointment where intentions may be misinterpreted.

B. Be meticulous about recordkeeping and documentation procedures. Record the details of each sedation experience for every patient in the treatment file.

C. Practice within the standard of care established by the profession. Use updated equipment with the O_2 fail-safe mechanism for safe delivery to the patient. Follow the steps for appropriate N_2O/O_2 administration using the method of titration. Use the recommended scavenging procedures for the sake of those exposed to trace gas contamination.

D. Be knowledgeable about the levels of sedation and be appropriately prepared to handle the next (deeper) level than that which you have intended. N_2O is a safe drug but it is your responsibility to know how to react in any given situation.

E. Maintain an adequate and current malpractice insurance policy.

F. Practice within the parameters of the discipline. Do not ask others to perform the procedure when they are not legally allowed to do so, and do not perform the task yourself if you are not permitted.

REFERENCE

1. American Dental Association: *Guidelines for the use of conscious sedation, deep sedation and general anesthesia for dentists*, Chicago, 2002, American Dental Association.

20
Commonly Asked Questions Regarding N_2O/O_2 Sedation

1. *Can I use oral premedication with N_2O/O_2?*
Yes, but remember there will be a synergistic effect between the N_2O and other drugs. Therefore it is important to know the pharmacology of all the drugs involved.

2. *Is it okay to eat before using N_2O/O_2?*
Yes, a light, nonfatty meal eaten no sooner than 2 hours before the procedure is fine. It is best to avoid heavy meals.

3. *Can an open flame be used in the operatory with N_2O?*
Yes, however, N_2O supports combustion. Therefore no open flame should be near compressed N_2O or O_2.

4. *Is a pulse oximeter necessary for N_2O/O_2 sedation?*
No, not if it is given in concentrations below 50%. Above this level, it is recommended to monitor the patient with a pulse oximeter.

5. *Is sickle cell anemia a contraindication to N_2O/O_2 use?*
No, in fact, preventive measures for sickle cell crisis use 100% O_2.

6. *Does the rubber hosing need to be sterilized after each patient?*
Any part of the rubber hosing that is not corrugated can be sterilized. This should be done after each patient.

7. *Can N_2O become addicting?*
N_2O can be addictive or habituating like most substances.

8. *How does N_2O affect the lactating (nursing) mother?*
N_2O has no effect on breast milk.

9. *Can N_2O/O_2 enhance difficult venipuncture?*
Yes, a short course of N_2O/O_2 can enhance venous distention and visibility.

10. *Can I go back to work right after I've used N_2O?*
Yes, there is a full and complete recovery following an adequate amount of 100% O_2 after a procedure.

11. *Can I use N₂O without O₂?*

No, the O_2 molecule must be available for human metabolism. Using N_2O without O_2 could result in death.

12. *Can any age group use N₂O/O₂?*

Yes, that is one of the attributes of N_2O.

13. *Does insurance pay for N₂O/O₂ sedation?*

Yes, some companies reimburse for this service although others do not. In the United States, the ADA reimbursement code is #09230.

14. *Can a person with asthma use N₂O/O₂ sedation?*

Absolutely, asthmatics do very well with N_2O.

15. *What is the number one potential negative side effect?*

There is the potential for nausea and vomiting, particularly if inappropriately high concentrations of N_2O are used or an inappropriate administration technique is used.

16. *Can N₂O be used with a laser present?*

Yes, this is not a contraindication for its use.

17. *Can a rash around the nose indicate an allergy to the nose piece (latex nasal hood)?*

Yes, if the individual is latex sensitive or if the nasal hood was inappropriately disinfected and not sterilized.

18. *Is it necessary to chart the N₂O/O₂ procedure?*

Yes, for legal reasons it is required to document each N_2O/O_2 procedure. A sample of a sedation record is included in Chapter 13 and in Appendix C.

19. *Where can I rent an IR spectrophotometer to measure trace gas N₂O in my office?*

An inexpensive and convenient way is to contact your local hospital or gas supplier.

20. *Is N₂O/O₂ sedation contraindicated for an individual with trisomy 21?*

No. N_2O/O_2 sedation is used for a variety of medically compromised patients.

21. *Is a back-up portable system necessary?*

It is highly recommended to have a second tank of each gas immediately available should one be emptied in the middle of a procedure.

22. *Can you give oxycodone (Vicodin) with N₂O/O₂ sedation?*

The patient is completely recovered from N_2O/O_2 sedation. Any postoperative medication will have no interaction with the previous N_2O/O_2 experience.

23. *What does it mean when the reservoir bag collapses (sticks)?*
It may mean the valve in the mask is missing and a new nasal hood needs to be placed.

24. *Is a written consent form necessary?*
Certainly verbal consent must be obtained before each N$_2$O/O$_2$ procedure. A sample written consent form has been provided in Appendix D.

25. *Why is the N$_2$O/O$_2$ machine such an important piece of emergency equipment?*
N$_2$O/O$_2$ sedation machines allow for positive-pressure O$_2$ to be delivered to the patient. This is the treatment for laryngospasm and ensuring the lungs are well ventilated with O$_2$. It also does not require the skill associated with using an Ambu bag.

21
Future Trends in N$_2$O/O$_2$ Sedation

Fortunately, advances in medical technology have allowed people to live longer, more productive lives. However, there is still a critical need for healthcare services and unfortunately, not enough professionals to provide those services. Access to care has become a focus of many healthcare disciplines. Accommodating all people and their healthcare needs will be a subject of study well into the future.

Inhalation sedation using N$_2$O/O$_2$ for pain and anxiety management is being enhanced in many ways. Several disciplines are already broadening their scope of practice to allow additional professionals to administer N$_2$O/O$_2$ sedation. Within the United States, certification is required to ensure personnel are well trained and knowledgeable about the use of N$_2$O/O$_2$ and the appropriate technique for administration. There are a growing number of continuing education courses being offered both nationally and internationally on this subject. It is important to continue to emphasize its importance in academic institutions, in continuing education courses, and as part of national and international conferences to provide a future for N$_2$O/O$_2$ use.

It is the duty of practitioners to become involved with those agencies and individuals who are responsible for safe products and safe procedures. We have faith that the manufacturers of N$_2$O/O$_2$ equipment will provide you and your patients with the highest quality products available and will continue to pursue technological avenues for minimizing trace gas contamination. There is no doubt that the industry will continue its dedication to providing quality equipment for the safe delivery of N$_2$O and O$_2$.

Market predictions indicate an increase in the consumption of N$_2$O. Patients will continue to undergo surgical procedures at an increasing rate. Healthcare will always be a priority. N$_2$O/O$_2$ sedation will be a useful part of that future. The future is bright and we are excited to be a part of it. In spite of all these attributes and overall growth, there is suspicion in some parts of the world and restrictions are being placed on the use of N$_2$O and O$_2$ from simple ignorance and lack of training. It is our mission to inform others and bring this useful product to the patients who need it.

APPENDIXES

A
Manufacturers and Organizational Resources

Authors

Morris Clark, DDS, FACD
Department of Oral and Maxillofacial Surgery
University of Colorado Health Sciences Center
4200 East 9th Street
Denver, CO 80262
Telephone: 303-315-6345
Fax: 303-315-0336
morris.clark@uchsc.edu

Ann Brunick, RDH, MS
Department of Dental Hygiene
University of South Dakota
120 East Hall/414 East Clark Street
Vermillion, SD 57069
Telephone: 605-677-5379
Fax: 605-677-5638
abrunick@usd.edu

N_2O/O_2 Equipment Manufacturers

Accutron, Inc.
2020 West Melinda Lane
Phoenix, AZ 85027
Telephone: 800-531-2221
Fax: 602-780-0444
accutron-inc.com

Matrx Medical Inc.
145 Med County Drive
Orchard Park, NY 14127
Telephone: 800-847-1000
Fax: 716-662-7130
matrxmedical.com

Porter Instrument Co., Inc.
245 Township Line Road, Box 907
Hatfield, PA 19440-0907
Telephone: 800-457-2001
Fax: 215-723-2199
porterinst.com

Personal Monitoring Devices

Advanced Chemical Sensor, Inc.
3201 North Dixie Highway
Boca Raton, FL 33431
Telephone: 561-338-3116
Fax: 561-338-5737
acsbadges.com

Assay Technology
1070 East Meadow Circle
Palo Alto, CA 94303-4230
Telephone: 800-833-1258
assaytec.com

Kem Medical Products Corp.
14 Engineers Lane
Farmingdale, NY 11735
Telephone: 800-553-0330
Fax: 631-454-8083
kemmed.com

Medical Safety Systems, Inc.
565 White Pond Drive
Akron, OH 44320
Telephone: 888-803-9303
Fax: 330-865-4393
ms2info.com

Nevin Laboratories, Inc.
5000 South Halsted Street
Chicago, IL 60609
Telephone: 800-544-5337
Fax: 773-624-7337
nevinlabs.com

IR Spectrophotometry

Bacharach, Inc.
625 Alpha Drive
Pittsburgh, PA 15238
Telephone: 800-736-4666 US
Telephone: 800-328-5217 Canada
bacharach-inc.com

Thermo Environmental Instruments, Inc.
27 Forge Parkway
Franklin, MA 02038
Telephone: 508-553-6861
Fax: 508-520-1460
thermo.com/tei

Electronic Micromanometer

Shortridge Instruments, Inc.
7855 East Redfield Road
Scottsdale, AZ 85260
Telephone: 480-991-6744
Fax: 480-443-1267
shortridge.com

Organizational Resources

American Conference of Government Industrial Hygienists
1330 Kemper Meadow Drive, Suite 600
Cincinnati, OH 45240
Telephone: 513-742-2020
Fax: 513-742-3355
acgih.org

American Dental Association
211 East Chicago Avenue
Chicago, IL 60611
Telephone: 800-621-8099
Fax: 312-440-7494
ada.org

American Dental Hygienists' Association
444 North Michigan Avenue, Suite 3400
Chicago, IL 60611
Telephone: 312-440-8900
Fax: 312-440-8929
adha.org

American Dental Society of Anesthesiology
211 East Chicago Avenue, Suite 780
Chicago, IL 60611
Telephone: 800-722-7788
Fax: 312-642-9713
adsahome.org

American Medical Association
515 North State Street
Chicago, IL 60611
Telephone: 312-464-5000
Fax: 312-464-4184
ama-assn.org

American Society of Anesthesiologists
520 North Northwest Highway
Park Ridge, IL 60068-2573
Telephone: 847-825-5586
Fax: 847-825-1692
asahq.org

Centers for Disease Control (CDC)
1600 Clifton Road Northeast
Atlanta, GA 30333
Telephone: 800-311-3435
cdc.gov

Compressed Gas Association, Inc.
4221 Walney Road, Fifth Floor
Chantilly, VA 20151-2923
Telephone: 703-788-2700
Fax: 703-961-1831
cganet.com

Gases and Welding Distributors Association
1900 Arch Street
Philadelphia, PA 19103
Telephone: 215-564-3484
Fax: 215-963-9784
gawda.org

National Fire Protection Association
1 Batterymarch Park, Box 9101
Quincy, MA 02269-9101
Telephone: 617-770-3000
Fax: 617-770-0700
nfpa.org

National Inspection Testing Certification (ITC)
501 Shatto Place, Suite 200
Los Angeles, CA 90020
Telephone: 877-457-6482
ppe.org

National Institute for Occupational Safety and Health (NIOSH)
4676 Columbia Parkway
Cincinnati, OH 45226
Telephone: 800-356-4674
Fax: 513-533-8573
cdc.gov/niosh

Occupational Safety and Health Administration (OSHA)
Health Standards Programs
United States Department of Labor
200 Constitution Avenue Northwest
Washington, DC 20210
Telephone: 800-321-6742
osha.gov

Piping, Industry, Progress, and Education (PIPE)
501 Shatto Place, Suite 200
Los Angeles, CA 90020
Telephone: 800-457-7473
Fax: 213-382-2501
pipe.org

B
Percent of N_2O/O_2 Administered*

LITERS PER MINUTE N_2O	0.5	1	1.5	2	2.5	3	3.5	4	4.5	5
0.5	50%	33%	25%	20%	17%	14%	13%	11%	10%	9%
1	67%	50%	40%	33%	29%	25%	22%	20%	18%	17%
1.5	75%	60%	50%	43%	38%	33%	30%	27%	25%	23%
2	80%	67%	57%	50%	44%	40%	36%	33%	31%	29%
2.5	83%	71%	63%	56%	50%	45%	42%	38%	36%	33%
3	86%	75%	67%	60%	55%	50%	46%	43%	40%	38%
3.5	88%	78%	70%	64%	58%	54%	50%	47%	44%	41%
4	89%	80%	73%	67%	62%	57%	53%	50%	47%	44%
4.5	90%	82%	75%	69%	64%	60%	56%	53%	50%	47%
5	91%	83%	77%	71%	67%	63%	59%	56%	53%	50%
5.5	92%	85%	79%	73%	69%	65%	61%	58%	55%	52%
6	92%	86%	80%	75%	71%	67%	63%	60%	57%	55%
6.5	93%	87%	81%	76%	72%	68%	65%	62%	59%	57%
7	93%	88%	82%	78%	74%	70%	67%	64%	61%	58%
7.5	94%	88%	83%	79%	75%	71%	68%	65%	63%	60%
8	94%	89%	84%	80%	76%	73%	70%	67%	64%	62%
8.5	94%	89%	85%	81%	77%	74%	71%	68%	65%	63%
9	95%	90%	86%	82%	78%	75%	72%	69%	67%	64%
9.5	95%	90%	86%	83%	79%	76%	73%	70%	68%	66%
10	95%	91%	87%	83%	80%	77%	74%	71%	69%	67%

LITERS PER

*Greater than 70% N_2O administered exceeds the amount able to be delivered by sedation machine.

MINUTE O$_2$

5.5	6	6.5	7	7.5	8	8.5	9	9.5	10
8%	8%	7%	7%	6%	6%	6%	5%	5%	5%
15%	14%	13%	13%	12%	11%	11%	10%	10%	9%
21%	20%	19%	18%	17%	16%	15%	14%	14%	13%
27%	25%	24%	22%	21%	20%	19%	18%	17%	17%
31%	29%	28%	26%	25%	24%	23%	22%	21%	20%
35%	33%	32%	30%	29%	27%	26%	25%	24%	23%
39%	37%	35%	33%	32%	30%	29%	28%	27%	26%
42%	40%	38%	36%	35%	33%	32%	31%	30%	29%
45%	43%	41%	39%	38%	36%	35%	33%	32%	31%
48%	45%	43%	42%	40%	38%	37%	36%	34%	33%
50%	48%	46%	44%	42%	41%	39%	38%	37%	35%
52%	50%	48%	46%	44%	43%	41%	40%	39%	38%
54%	52%	50%	48%	46%	45%	43%	42%	41%	39%
56%	54%	52%	50%	48%	47%	45%	44%	42%	41%
58%	56%	54%	52%	50%	48%	47%	45%	44%	43%
59%	57%	55%	53%	52%	50%	48%	47%	46%	44%
61%	59%	57%	55%	53%	52%	50%	49%	47%	46%
62%	60%	58%	56%	55%	53%	51%	50%	49%	47%
63%	61%	59%	58%	56%	54%	53%	51%	50%	49%
65%	63%	61%	59%	57%	56%	54%	53%	51%	50%

C

N_2O/O_2 Sedation Record

Date:_____ Patient Name:_____ Age:_____

ASA Classification: I   II   III   IV

Indications for N_2O/O_2:_____

Procedural Data:

	PREOPERATIVE	INTRAOPERATIVE (Moderate Sedation)	POSTOPERATIVE
Blood pressure:	_____	_____	_____
Pulse:	_____	_____	_____
Respiration:	_____	_____	_____
Spo_2 (moderate sedation):	_____	_____	_____

Tidal volume (L/min):_____   Peak % N_2O adm:_____

Postop 100% O_2:   _____ minutes

Recovery (pt comments):_____

Adverse Reactions/Comments:

Clinician's signature:_____

D
Informed Consent for N_2O/O_2 Sedation

I understand that my treatment today will include the procedure of N_2O/O_2 administration.

I, _____, have been informed of the purpose of the procedure and how it will benefit my treatment. The procedure has been described to me and I understand how it will be accomplished. I should feel more relaxed and less anxious.

I understand that certain risk(s) may be associated with this procedure, such as headache, dizziness, nausea, and vomiting. Some patients at high levels of N_2O can experience dreaming and hallucinations. I understand the risk(s) associated with this procedure and I further understand the risk(s) that may occur if the procedure is not completed.

I also realize that my doctor must know if I have taken any type of medication or drugs within the past seventy-two (72) hours because these may cause an adverse reaction when N_2O/O_2 is administered. I verify that I have told my doctor about any such medications and drugs.

I have been informed of the alternatives to N_2O/O_2 sedation and their associated risks.

All of my questions and concerns have been satisfactorily answered and addressed.

Therefore, I give my informed consent to the administration of N_2O/O_2 sedation and agree to hold harmless, release, and indemnify agents, servants, students, and employees of the office/clinic of _____ from any and all causes of action, claims, demands, or liability that may arise out of such treatment on behalf of myself, my heirs, my executors, administrators or assigns; or on behalf of my minor child or children or his/her (their) heirs, executors, administrators or assigns.

Signed:_____   Date:_____

Witness:_____   Date:_____

E

Overview of Administration of N_2O/O_2 Sedation

1. Inspect all N_2O/O_2 equipment for proper setup. Periodically check pressure connections with a soap and water solution per manufacturer's recommendations. Inspect the tubing and reservoir bag for cracks or tears.
2. Confirm the adequacy of all scavenging methods to include the vacuum exhaust and ventilation for the area.
3. Review the patient's health history and record vital signs. Obtain informed consent.
4. Activate O_2 flow, fit nasal hood or face mask, and establish appropriate tidal volume. Observe reservoir bag.
5. Initiate N_2O flow and titrate appropriately while constantly assessing the patient.
6. Upon termination of the N_2O, begin a minimum postoperative oxygenation period of 5 minutes.
7. Assess the patient for appropriate recovery. Administer additional O_2 if necessary.
8. Document the procedure appropriately in the patient's file (i.e., sedation record).
9. Properly disassemble and disinfect equipment.

F
Health Insurance Portability and Accountability Act (HIPAA) of 1996

The Health Insurance Portability and Accountability Act (HIPAA) of 1996 was signed into law by President Bill Clinton on August 21, 1996. Conclusive regulations were issued on August 17, 2000, to be instated by October 16, 2002. HIPAA requires that the transactions of all patient health care information be formatted in a standardized electronic style. In addition to protecting the privacy and security of patient information, HIPAA includes legislation on the formation of medical savings accounts, the authorization of a fraud and abuse control program, the easy transport of health insurance coverage, and the simplification of administrative terms and conditions.

HIPAA encompasses three primary areas, and its privacy requirements can be broken down into three types—privacy standards, patients' rights, and administrative requirements.

1. **Privacy Standards.** A central concern of HIPAA is the careful use and disclosure of protected health information (PHI), which generally is electronically controlled health information that is able to be distinguished individually. PHI also refers to verbal communication although the HIPAA Privacy Rule is not intended to hinder necessary verbal communication. The U.S. Department of Health and Human Services (USDHHS) does not require restructuring, such as soundproofing, architectural changes, and so forth, but some caution is necessary when exchanging health information by conversation.

   An Acknowledgment of Receipt Notice of Privacy Practices, which allows patient information to be used or divulged for treatment, payment, or health care operations (TPO), should be procured from each patient. A detailed and time-sensitive authorization can also be issued, which allows the dentist to release information in special circumstances other than TPOs. A *written consent* is also an option. Dentists can disclose PHI *without* acknowledgement, consent, or authorization in very special situations, for example, perceived child abuse, public health supervision, fraud investigation, or law enforcement with valid permission (i.e., a warrant). When divulging PHI, a dentist must try to disclose only the *minimum necessary* information, to help safeguard the patient's information as much as possible.

Data from *HIPAA Privacy Kit* and http://www.ada.org/prof/prac/issues/topics/hipaa/index.html. (From *Mosby's Dental Dictionary*, St Louis, Mosby, 2004.)

It is important that dental professionals adhere to HIPAA standards because health care providers (as well as health care clearinghouses and health care plans) who convey *electronically* formatted health information via an outside billing service or merchant are considered *covered entities.* Covered entities may be dealt serious civil and criminal penalties for violation of HIPAA legislation. Failure to comply with HIPAA privacy requirements may result in civil penalties of up to $100 per offense with an annual maximum of $25,000 for repeated failure to comply with the same requirement. Criminal penalties resulting from the illegal mishandling of private health information can range from $50,000 and/or 1 year in prison to $250,000 and/or 10 years in prison.

2. **Patients' Rights.** HIPAA allows patients, authorized representatives, and parents of minors, as well as minors, to become more aware of the health information privacy to which they are entitled. These rights include, but are not limited to, the right to view and copy their health information, the right to dispute alleged breaches of policies and regulations, and the right to request alternative forms of communicating with their dentist. If any health information is released for any reason other than TPO, the patient is entitled to an account of the transaction. Therefore, it is important for dentists to keep accurate records of such information and to provide them when necessary.

   The HIPAA Privacy Rule determines that the parents of a minor have access to their child's health information. This privilege may be overruled, for example, in cases where there is suspected child abuse or the parent consents to a term of confidentiality between the dentist and the minor. The parents' rights to access their child's PHI also may be restricted in situations when a legal entity, such as a court, intervenes and when a law does not require a parent's consent. For a full list of patient rights provided by HIPAA, be sure to acquire a copy of the law and to understand it well.

3. **Administrative Requirements.** Complying with HIPAA legislation may seem like a chore, but it does not need to be so. It is recommended that you become appropriately familiar with the law, organize the requirements into simpler tasks, begin compliance early, and document your progress in compliance. An important first step is to evaluate the current information and practices of your office.

   Dentists will need to write a *privacy policy* for their office, a document for their patients detailing the office's practices concerning PHI. The ADA's *HIPAA Privacy Kit* includes forms that you (the dentist) can use to customize your privacy policy. It is useful to try to understand the role of health care information for your patients and the ways in which they deal with the information while they are visiting your office. Train your staff; make sure they are familiar with the terms of HIPAA and your office's privacy policy and related forms. HIPAA requires that you designate a *privacy officer,* a person in your office who will be responsible for applying the new policies in your office, fielding complaints, and making choices involving the minimum necessary requirements. Another person with the role of *contact person* will process complaints.

A *Notice of Privacy Practices*—a document detailing the patient's rights and the dental office's obligations concerning PHI—also must be drawn up. Further, any role of a third party with access to PHI must be clearly documented. This third party is known as a *business associate* (BA) and is defined as any entity who, on behalf of the dentist, takes part in any activity that involves exposure of PHI. The *HIPAA Privacy Kit* provides a copy of the USD-HHS "Business Associate Contract Terms," which provides a concrete format for detailing BA interactions.

The main HIPAA privacy compliance date, including all staff training, was April 14, 2003, although many covered entities who submitted a request and a compliance plan by October 15, 2002, were granted one-year extensions. Contact your local branch of the ADA for details. It is recommended that dentists prepare their offices ahead of time for all deadlines, which include preparing privacy polices and forms, business associate contracts, and employee training sessions.

For a comprehensive discussion of all of these terms and requirements, a complete list of HIPAA policies and procedures, and a full collection of HIPAA privacy forms, contact the American Dental Association for a *HIPAA Privacy Kit*. The relevant ADA Web site is www.ada.org/goto/hipaa. Other Web sites that may contain useful information about HIPAA are as follows:

- USDHHS Office of Civil Rights www.hhs.gov/ocr/hipaa
- Work Group on Electronic Data Interchange www.wedi.org/SNIP
- Phoenix Health www.hipaadvisory.com
- USDHHS Office of the Assistant Secretary for Planning and Evaluation http://aspe.os.dhhs.gov/admnsimp/

G
Overview of CDC Hand Hygiene Guidelines*

The CDC recently released new recommendations for hand hygiene in healthcare settings. Hand hygiene is a term that applies to either handwashing, use of an antiseptic hand rub, or surgical hand antisepsis. Evidence suggests that hand antisepsis, the cleansing of hands with an antiseptic hand rub, is more effective in reducing nosocomial infections than plain handwashing.

Follow these guidelines in the care of all patients:

- Continue to wash hands with either a nonantimicrobial or an antimicrobial soap and water whenever the hands are visibly soiled.
- Use an alcohol-based hand rub to routinely decontaminate the hands in the following clinical situations: (*Note:* If alcohol-based hand rubs are not available, the alternative is hand washing.)
  - Before and after client contact
  - Before donning sterile gloves when inserting central intravascular catheters
  - Before performing nonsurgical invasive procedures (e.g., urinary catheter insertion, nasotracheal suctioning)
  - After contact with body fluids or excretions, mucous membranes, nonintact skin, and wound dressings
  - If moving from a contaminated body site (rectal area or mouth) to a clean body site (surgical wound, urinary meatus) during client care
  - After contact with inanimate objects (including medical equipment) in the immediate vicinity of the client
  - After removing gloves
- Before eating and after using a restroom, wash hands with a nonantimicrobial or an antimicrobial soap and water.
- Antimicrobial-impregnated wipes (i.e., towelettes) are not a substitute for using an alcohol-based hand rub or antimicrobial soap.
- If exposure to *Bacillus anthracis* is suspected or proven, wash hands with a nonantimicrobial or an antimicrobial soap and water. The physical action of washing and rinsing hands is recommended because alcohols, chlorhexidine, iodophors, and other antiseptic agents have poor activity against spores.

---

*Modified from Centers for Disease Control and Prevention: *MMWR* 51(RR16):1, 2002. www.cdc.gov/handhygiene

Method for Decontaminating Hands

When using an alcohol-based hand rub, apply product to palm of one hand and rub hands together, covering all surfaces of hands and fingers, until hands are dry. Follow the manufacturer's recommendations regarding the volume of product to use.

Follow these guidelines for surgical hand antisepsis:
- Surgical hand antisepsis reduces the resident microbial count on the hands to a minimum.
- The CDC recommends using an antimicrobial soap, and to scrub hands and forearms for the length of time recommended by the manufacturer, usually 2 to 6 minutes. The Association of Operating Room Nurses recommends 5 to 10 minutes. Refer to agency policy for time required.
- When using an alcohol-based surgical hand-scrub product with persistent activity, follow the manufacturer's instructions. Before applying the alcohol solution, prewash hands and forearms with a nonantimicrobial soap and dry hands and forearms completely. After application of the alcohol-based product as recommended, allow hands and forearms to dry thoroughly before donning sterile gloves.

General recommendations for hand hygiene:
- Use hand lotions or creams to minimize the occurrence of irritant contact dermatitis associated with hand antisepsis or handwashing.
- Do not wear artificial fingernails or extenders when having direct contact with clients at high risk (e.g., those in intensive-care units or operating rooms).
- Keep natural nails tips less than 1/4-inch long.
- Wear gloves when contact with blood or other potentially infectious materials, mucous membranes, and nonintact skin could occur.
- Remove gloves after caring for a client. Do not wear the same pair of gloves for the care of more than one client, and do not wash gloves between uses with different clients.
- Change gloves during client care if moving from a contaminated body site to a clean body site.

INDEX*

A

Abscess(es)
  incising, 151
  liver, drainage of, 156
Abuse
inhalant, 185–187. *See also* Inhalant
  abuse
of nitrous oxide, 185–194. *See also*
  Nitrous oxide, abuse of;
  Recreational use of nitrous
  oxide
Accutron, 49, 62f, 64, 64f
Acupressure, 24
Acupuncture, 24
Acute myocardial infarction. *See*
  Myocardial infarction
ADA. *See* American Dental Association
  (ADA)
Addiction, withdrawal from, 156
Addictive potential, of nitrous oxide,
  201
Adolescents, inhalant abuse by,
  185–186
Adrenal dysfunction, 93
Age, nitrous oxide/oxygen sedation and,
  202
AIDS/HIV, 92
Air ambulances, 38
Air inlet, emergency, 69
Air Liquide America, 43
Airway
  obstruction of, in moderate
    sedation, management of,
    86–87
  preprocedure assessment of, 102,
    194b
Alarms, 69

Alcohol
  addiction to, withdrawal from, 156
  intoxication with, nitrous oxide
    contraindicated in, 96
Allergy(ies), 95
  drug, preventing reactions from, 108
  latex, nasal hoods and, 202
Altitudes, high, 38
Alveolar ducts, anatomy of, 80f, 81
Alveolar sacs, anatomy of, 81
Alveolar ventilation, 82
Alveoli, anatomy of, 81
Alzheimer's disease, 95
Ambient air, monitoring of, 174, 180
Ambulances, 38, 151, 152f
Ambulatory foot surgery, 154
American Dental Association (ADA),
    position statement of, on maximum
    nitrous exposure limit, 172
American Society of Anesthesiologists
    (ASA)
  classification of, for patient medical
    risk, 100–101, 101b
  Practice Guidelines for Sedation and
    Analgesia by Non-
    Anesthesiologists, 4
Ammonium nitrate, in nitrous oxide
    manufacturing, 41
Amnestic properties, 158
Amyl nitrite, 186
Analgesics, sites of action of, 18f
Anatomic dead space, 82
Andrews, Edmund, 13
Anemia, 92
  megaloblastic, 173
  sickle cell, nitrous oxide/oxygen
    sedation and, 201

*Page numbers followed by *b* refer to boxes; *f,* figures; *t,* tables.

Anesthesia
  electronic dental, 24
  evolution of, 10–15
  general, 25
    definition of, 22
  inhalation, 39, 39b
  local, 14, 24
    administered with nitrous
      oxide/oxygen sedation, 31
    potency of, 38–39
Angina pectoris, 90
Antidepressants, nitrous oxide
  contraindicated with, 96
Anxiety
  acknowledgment of, 20
  assessment of, 20, 21f, 99–100
  definition of, 19–20
  management of. See Pain/anxiety
    management
  questions about, 99–100
Anxiolysis, definition of, 21
Aortoperipheral arteriography, 156
Arteriography, visceral, 156
Arteriosclerosis, 90
Arthroplasty, digital, 154
Arthroscopy, temporomandibular joint,
  bilateral, 156
ASA. See American Society of
  Anesthesiologists
Asphyxial death from recreational
  nitrous oxide use, 191–192
Aspiration, 91
  in oversedation, 117
  of vomitus in moderate sedation,
    management of, 87
Asthma, 91
  nitrous oxide/oxygen sedation and,
    202
Atherosclerosis, 90
Atmospheric gas, composition of,
  82–83, 84b
Audioanalgesia, combined with nitrous
  oxide/oxygen sedation, 31
Autism, 95
Autoerotic asphyxial death, from
  recreational nitrous oxide use,
  192
Automobile accidents, from nitrous
  oxide abuse, 189
Automobile racing industry, nitrous
  oxide in, 43, 187

Awareness
  in appropriate minimal sedation,
    113–114
  in oversedation, 116

B

Barbiturates, nitrous oxide interacting
  with, 96
Baskett, Peter, 149, 150
Bert, Paul, 13
Bilateral temporomandibular joint
  arthroscopy, 156
Biliary catheter placement, 156
Biliary stone retrieval, 156
Biliary ureterastent placement, 156
Biohazards. See Health hazards
Biopsies, 151
  percutaneous, 156
Bladder bag, 49
Bleeding diastheses, 90
Bleomycin sulfate, 96
Blood flow, nitrous oxide effect on, 89
Blood-gas partition coefficient, 35
Blood pressure
  monitoring of, 101, 125, 128f
  nitrous oxide effect on, 89
  postoperative, 145
Body movement
  in appropriate minimal sedation,
    111
  in oversedation, 116
Bone marrow, megaloblastic changes
  in, from nitrous oxide exposure,
  92
Bowel obstruction, nitrous oxide
  contraindicated in, 93
Breast milk, nitrous oxide and,
  201
Breathing
  monitoring of, 134
  physiology of, 81–86
Breathing apparatus, 61–62f, 61–63
  selection of, 125
Breathing zone, personal, monitoring
  of, 180
Bronchi, anatomy of, 80–81, 80f
Bronchioli, anatomy of, 81
Bronchitis, chronic, 91, 92
Bunionectomy, 154
Burns, dressing, 151
Butyl nitrite, 186

C

Cancer, 95, 159
Car accidents, from nitrous oxide abuse, 189
Cardiac output, nitrous oxide effect on, 89
Cardiovascular system, 89–90
Carina, anatomy of, 80, 81f
Cataract surgery, 154
Catheter
  biliary, placement of, 156
  hepatic artery, placement of, 156
Catheterization, 151
Central gas supply system, 50–53, 50f, 51f, 52f, 53f
  piping system, 51, 53
  postoperative preparation, 137
  vs. portable gas supply system, 65–66, 71–73, 72t
Central nervous system (CNS), 90
  depressants of, in inhalant abuse, 186
Central-system manifold, 50–51, 50f, 51f
Cerebral blood flow, nitrous oxide effect on, 90
Cerebral palsy, 94
Cerebrovascular accident (stroke), 90
Chaperones, for nitrous oxide administration, 200
Chemical dependency, 95
Chemical industry, nitrous oxide in, 41
Chemical peeling, 153
Children
  anxiety of, 29
  audioanalgesia in, 31
  development of, 163, 164t
  in emergency departments, 150–151
  inhalant abuse by, 185–186
  nitrous oxide/oxygen sedation in, 158, 163–168. See also Pediatrics, nitrous oxide/oxygen sedation in
  oxygen l/min for, 126
Chloroform, evolution of, 11
Cholangiography, percutaneous, 156
Chronic obstructive pulmonary disease (COPD), 91
Cirrhosis, 93
CNS. See Central nervous system (CNS)
Cognition
  assessment of, 145
  nitrous oxide effect on, 171
Colt, Samuel, 7

Colton, Gardner, 9, 185
Compression, heat of, 33
Concentration effect, 36, 37f
Conduction tubing, 60–61, 60f
  inspection of, 119, 183
  sterilization/disinfection of, 140, 141f
Congenital heart disease, 90
Conscious sedation. See also Intravenous conscious sedation
Consent, informed, 97, 118, 198, 203, 214
  for pediatric patients, 168
Cooley, Samuel, 9
COPD. See Chronic obstructive pulmonary disease (COPD)
Correction fluid, inhalant abuse and, 186
Costs
  of nitrous oxide/oxygen sedation equipment, 65–66
  of nitrous oxide/oxygen sedation production, 43
  of nitrous oxide/oxygen sedation use, 71–74
Cryosurgery, 155
Curare, evolution of, 14
Cyclopropane, evolution of, 14
Cyst removal, 151
Cystic fibrosis, 92

D

Davy, Humphrey, 6–7, 185
Death, from inhalant abuse, 187
Delivery, labor and, 152–153
Dentistry, 157–158
  pediatric, nitrous oxide/oxygen sedation in, 163–164
Deoxyuridine suppression test, 173
Department of Transportation (DOT) regulations, for nitrous oxide packaging and transportation, 43
Dephlogisticated air, 6
Dephlogisticated nitrous air, 6
Depression, 155
Dermatology, 153
Desflurane, 39
Diabetes, 93
Diazepam, administered with nitrous oxide/oxygen sedation, 31
Diffusion hypoxia, 84, 86
  prevention of, 86

Digital arthrodesis, 154
Digital arthroplasty, 154
Digital sensor, 84, 85f
Dinitrogen monoxide, 33. *See also*
   Nitrous oxide
Discharge, following moderate sedation,
   guidelines for, 147
Disinfection, 138–140, 139f
Distraction techniques
   combined with nitrous oxide/oxygen
      sedation, 30
   in fear/anxiety management, 24
Documentation, 119, 140–141, 142b,
   143f, 200, 202
   of nitrous oxide/oxygen
      administration, 141, 142b, 143f,
      200
   of nitrous oxide/oxygen sedation,
      141, 142b, 143f
Dosimetry, time-weighted average, in
   personal monitoring, 175, 176f
DOT. *See* Department of Transportation
   (DOT)
Drawing test, during recovery, 146
Dreams, in oversedation, 116
Dressing burns, 151
Driving simulation test, during recovery,
   146
Drug allergies, 95
Drug intoxication, nitrous oxide
   contraindicated in, 96
Drug potency, determination of, 39
Drug testing, and nitrous oxide
   detection, 189
Dynorphins, 17

E

Ear, nose, and throat infections, 94
Eating, before nitrous oxide/oxygen
   sedation, 119, 201
Economic benefits of nitrous
   oxide/oxygen sedation, 70–74
EDA. *See* Electronic dental anesthesia
   (EDA)
Education
   of health personnel, 181, 182b,
      198–199
   for nitrous oxide/oxygen
      administration, 198–199
   of patients. *See* Patient instruction(s)
EEG. *See* Electroencephalogram (EEG)

Eger, Edmond, 89
Electroencephalogram (EEG), nitrous
   oxide effect on, 90
Electronic dental anesthesia (EDA), 24
   combined with nitrous oxide/oxygen
      sedation, 31
Emergence. *See* Recovery
Emergency medicine
   early patient stabilization in, 149,
      150, 150f
   nitrous oxide/oxygen sedation in,
      149–152, 203
      for children, 164–165
      clinical studies of, 150–151
      current use in, 150–151
      equipment for, 151, 152f
      historical use in, 149–150
      indications for, 151
      products of, 152
Emergency preparedness, 106
Empathy toward patients by health
   professionals, 20
Emphysema, 91, 92
Endocrine system, 92–93
Endorphins, 17
Endoscopy, gastrointestinal, 155–156
   nitrous oxide/oxygen sedation in, for
      children, 165
Enflurane, 39
Enkephalins, 17
Entonox, 152
Environmental monitoring, 180
Epiglottis, 78, 79f
Equipment, sedation
   in ambulances, 151
   back-up portable system, 202
   with capability of mixing gases, 63,
      64f
   cost of, 65–66
   customization of, 65
   design of, 63–65, 64–65f
   disinfection of, 138–140, 139f
   with electronic digital display, 63–64,
      65f
   emergency, 106
   maintenance of, 66, 183
   safety features of, 66–69, 67–68f
   with separate gas flow controls, 63,
      64f
   sterilization of, 138–140, 141–142f
   variations in, 63–66

Ether, evolution of, 10–11
Ether dome, 10, 11f
Ethics, 193–194, 199–200
Euphoria, from nitrous oxide, 6, 192
Evacuation system, 178, 180
Exhaust register louvers, 180
Expiration, 82
Eye(s)
  in appropriate minimal sedation,
    111–112
  in oversedation, 116
  surgery on, 94–95, 156

F

Face mask, 61, 63
Facial expression
  in appropriate minimal sedati
    on, 112
  in oversedation, 116
Fail-safe mechanisms
  flowmeter, 56, 58, 59f
  oxygen, 49, 66, 200
Fainting spells, nitrous oxide effect
  on, 90
False vocal cords, anatomy of, 79
Fasting, preprocedure, 102, 105b
FDA. *See* Food and Drug Administration
  (FDA)
Fear
  acknowledgment of, 20
  assessment of, 20, 21f
  definition of, 20
  management of, 28–29
  pain interacting with, 20
Fetal abnormalities, 173, 190
Fixed-ratio self-administered
  equipment in emergency medicine,
  150
Flomenbaum, N, 150
Flowmeter, 55–56, 58–59f
  fail-safe mechanism for, 56, 58,
    59f
Flowmeter gas tubes, 50
Food and Drug Administration (FDA),
  regulations of, for nitrous oxide
  packaging, 43
Food industry, nitrous oxide in, 43
Foot surgery, ambulatory, 154
Fresh air exchange, 179–180
Frostbite, from recreational exposure to
  nitrous oxide, 191

G

Gas cylinders. *See also* Nitrous oxide
  cylinders; Oxygen cylinders
  for nitrous oxide/oxygen storage,
    43–49, 45f, 47f, 48f
  color coding of, 44, 46t
  longevity of, 44
  markings of, 44, 45f
  NFPA regulation of, 47
  safety of, 44, 46–47
  size of, 44, 47f
Gas exchange, in respiration, 83–84
Gas flow controls, 63, 64f
Gas supply system, central vs. portable,
  65–66, 71–73, 72t
Gastrointestinal system, 93
  endoscopy of, 155–156
  nitrous oxide/oxygen sedation in,
    for children, 165
General anesthesia, 25
Genitourinary/reproductive system,
  93–94
Grand Exhibition, 9
"Grocery store high," 189
Guidelines, for nitrous oxide
  administration, 4, 200
Gynecologic laparoscopy, 153

H

Hair transplantation, 153
Hallucinations, in oversedation, 116
Halothane, 39
  evolution of, 14
Hand/eye coordination exercise, during
  recovery, 146–147
Hand-held nitrous oxide monitoring
  device, 175–176, 179f
Hand hygiene guidelines, CDC,
  219–220
Head/facial injuries, nitrous oxide
  contraindicated during, 96
Head injuries, 151
Health care
  changing environment of, 70–71
  economics of, 70–71
Health hazards to health professionals
  from chronic nitrous oxide
    exposure, 171–182, 190–192
  biologic issues and, 172–173
  detection and monitoring in,
    174–176

Health hazards to health professionals
from chronic nitrous oxide
exposure—cont'd
health concerns and, 172–173
literature on
current, 173–174
historical, 171–172
Health history, 99–100
Health Insurance Portability and
Accountability Act of 1996,
216–218
Health professionals
attitude of, 118
chronic nitrous oxide exposure of,
potential biohazards of,
171–182. *See also* Health hazards
to health professionals from
chronic nitrous oxide exposure
education of, 181, 182b, 198–21
empathy toward patients, 20
and nitrous oxide abuse, 187, 192
avoidance of, 199
selection of, 70
sexual impropriety allegations
against, 192–193
avoidance of, 200
supply and demand of, 70–71
Heart murmur, 90
Heat of compression, 33
Hematopoietic system, 92
Hemophilia, 92
Hemorrhoid removal, 151
Hepatic artery catheter placement, 156
Hepatic system, 93
Hepatitis, 93
Hewitt, Fredrick, 49
High pressure lines, assessment of, 119
History, health, 99–100
HIV/AIDS, 92
Homemade nitrous oxide, for
recreational use, 188
Horace Wells experiment, 9–10
Hyperactivity, 155
Hypertension, 90
Hyperthermia, malignant, 95
Hypnosis
combined with nitrous oxide/oxygen
sedation, 30
in pain/anxiety management, 24
Hypnosuggestive properties, of nitrous
oxide/oxygen sedation, 158

Hypoxia, 91–92
diffusion, 84, 86
prevention of, 86
Hypoxic drive, nitrous oxide
contraindicated in, 91–92

I

Iatrosedation, 22, 24
Imagery, combined with nitrous oxide
oxygen sedation, 30
Implant surgery, ocular, 154
Incoherence, in oversedation, 116
Index safety system, 66–67, 67f
Individual biovariability, in
pain/anxiety management, 26
through titration, 108–109, 110, 135,
144
Industrial use, of nitrous oxide, 41–42
Infarction, myocardial, 90
Infections, upper respiratory tract,
nitrous oxide effect on, 90, 92
Informed consent, 97, 118, 198, 203
for pediatric patients, 168
Infrared spectrophotometry, 174–175,
175f, 180
equipment rental for, 202
Inhalant abuse, 185–187
central nervous system depressants
and, 186
in children and adolescents, 185–186
death from, 187
examples of, 186
inhaled products, availability of, 186
through occupational exposure, 186
Inhalation anesthesia, minimum
alveolar concentration for, 39, 39t
Inhalation sedation, 25
teaching of, in dental schools, 14
Inspiration, 81
Insufflation, 153
Insurance
malpractice, 200
for nitrous oxide/oxygen sedation,
202
Intracranial pressure, nitrous oxide
effect on, 90
Intramuscular sedation, 25
Intraoperative monitoring, 134
Intraoperative vital signs, 105
Intravenous conscious sedation, 25
Isoflurane, 39

J

Jaundice, 93
Joint, temporomandibular, bilateral,
   arthroscopy of, 156

K

Kidney disease, 94

L

Labor and delivery, 152–153
Labor pains, chloroform for, evolution
   of, 11
Lactation, nitrous oxide and, 201
Langa, Harry, 14
Laparoscopy, gynecologic, 153
Laryngopharynx, anatomy of, 78–79,
   78f
Larynx, anatomy of, 79, 79f
Laser, nitrous oxide and, 202
Latex allergy, nasal hoods and, 202
Legal aspects, of nitrous oxide/oxygen
   administration, 197–198
Legislation, 193–194, 197
Leukemia, 92
Leukopenia, from nitrous oxide
   exposure, 190
Lhermitte's sign, 191
Licensure, of nitrous oxide/oxygen
   administration, 197, 198
Lightweight cylinders, 44
Liposuction, 153
Liters flow per minute (l/min) of
   oxygen, 125–127, 128b, 129
Liver, 93
Liver abscess drainage, 156
Local anesthesia, 14, 24
   combined with nitrous oxide/oxygen
      sedation, 31
   evolution of, 14
Lower airway, anatomy of, 79–81, 79f,
   80f
Lung capacity, 82

M

MAC. *See* Minimum alveolar
   concentration (MAC)
Magnetic resonance imaging (MRI), 157
Malignant hyperthermia, 95
Malpractice insurance, 200
Manifold, central-system, 50–51, 50f,
   51f

Manufacturing
   of nitrous oxide, 41–43, 42f
   of nitrous oxide/oxygen equipment,
      41–43, 42f
Marijuana addiction, withdrawal from,
   156
Matrx Medical Inc., 49, 64, 67f, 151, 152f
Medical industry, nitrous oxide in, 41
Medical risk
   ASA classification of, 100–101, 101b
   ASA-I, 100, 101b
   ASA-II, 100, 101b
   ASA-III, 100, 101b
   ASA-IV, 100, 101b
   ASA-V, 100, 101b
   ASA-VI, 101, 101b
   assessment of, 100–101
Medications, nitrous oxide interactions
   with, 96
Medullary center, physiology of, 81
Megaloblastic anemia, 173
Megaloblastic bone marrow changes,
   from nitrous oxide exposure, 92
Megaloblastic hematopoiesis, 190
Memory, assessment of, 145
Menszer, Leonard F., 12
Mental illness, 95
Mental retardation, 95
Meperidine hydrochloride,
   administered with nitrous
   oxide/oxygen sedation, 31
Methemoglobinemia, 92
Methione synthase, nitrous oxide effect
   on, 172, 190
Middle ear disturbances, 94
Mind-altering conditions, 95, 96–97
Minimum alveolar concentration
   (MAC), of inhalation anesthesia,
   39, 39t
Minute ventilation, 82
Monitoring
   ambient air, 174, 180
   blood pressure, 101, 125, 128f
   of breathing, 134
   of environment, 180
   intraoperative, 105, 134
   nitrous oxide, 174–176, 180
   patient, 101–102, 105, 118, 125, 128f,
      136
   of personal breathing zone, 180
   personal devices for, 175–176

Monitoring—cont'd
of pulse, 101, 125, 128f
of respiration, 101–102, 125
titration, 134
of vital signs, 101–102
Mood
in appropriate minimal sedation, 111,
113f
assessment of, 145
Morphine, 17
comparison to nitrous oxide/oxygen
sedation, 28
Morton, William, 10
MRI. *See* Magnetic resonance imaging
(MRI)
Multiple sclerosis, 94
Muscular dystrophy, 94
Musculoskeletal injuries, 151
Music, combined with nitrous
oxide/oxygen sedation, of, 313
Myasthenia gravis, 94
Myeloneuropathy, 173
Myocardial infarction, 89, 90, 158–159
Myocardial ischemia, nitrous oxide
effect on, 89

N

Nail matricectomy, 154
Nalozone hydrochloride, 17
Narcon (naloxone hydrochloride), 17
Nasal hood(s), 61–62f, 61–63
latex allergy and, 202
for pediatric patients, 166
securing to patient, 126, 127f
single-patient use, 140, 142f
sterilization of, 140
Nasopharynx, anatomy of, 77, 78f
National Fire Protection Association
(NFPA), regulations of, for gas
cylinder storage, 47
National Institute for Occupational
Safety and Health (NIOSH),
guidelines of, on maximum nitrous
oxide exposure limit in dentistry,
172
Nausea, in oversedation, 116, 202
Nellcor Puritan Bennett, 43
Neuroleptic-induced akathisia, 160
Neurologic side effects, of chronic
exposure to nitrous oxide, 173,
190–191

Neurology, 160
Neuromuscular system, 94
Neuropathy, peripheral, 190, 191
Nevi, incising, 151
NFPA. *See* National Fire Protection
Association (NFPA)
Nicotine addiction, withdrawal from,
156
NIOSH. *See* National Institute for
Occupational Safety and Health
(NIOSH)
Nitronox Field Model, 152, 152f
Nitrous air, 6
Nitrous oxide
abuse of, 185–194. *See also*
Recreational use of nitrous oxide
in auto racing industry, 43, 187
automobile accidents and, 189
avoidance of, 199
addictive nature of, 193
addictive potential of, 201
in atmosphere, 34
availability of, for recreational use,
187–188
blood-gas partition coefficient, 35
boiling point of, 33
chronic exposure to, health hazards
of, 190–192
in health professionals, 171–182.
See also Health hazards to
health professionals from
chronic nitrous oxide exposure
at college social activities, 187
concentration effect of, 36, 37f
contraindications to, 91–92, 91b, 94,
96
cost of, 73, 73f
cylinders of, 43–47, 45f, 47f, 48f, 49
pressure gauge reading of, 47, 48f,
49
dangers of, 33
desirable characteristics of, 29b
detection in routine urine tests, 189
effects of solubility on, 35
effects on opioid system, 17
ethical issues and, 193–194, 199–200
euphoric effects of, 6, 192
evacuation flow rate of, 174
by health professionals, 187, 192
at high altitudes, 38
homemade, for recreational use, 188

Nitrous oxide—cont'd
  idiosyncratic reactions to, 109
  inhalation, history of, 6–8
  interaction with body systems and
    conditions, 89–95
  lactation and, 201
  laser and, 202
  leaks of, 177–178, 178f, 179f, 180
    prevention of, 180
  manufacturing of, 41–43, 42f
  maximum exposure limit of, 172
  metabolism of, 38
  minimum alveolar concentration for,
    39, 39t
  molecular weight of, 33
  monitoring of, 174–176, 180
  neurologic side effects of, 173,
    190–191
  optimal flow rate for, 178
  overexposure to, prevention of,
    180–181, 182b
  oxygen and, 202
  packaging of, 43–49, 44f, 45f, 46t,
    47f, 48f
    regulatory control of, 43
  partial pressure gradients of, 35–36,
    36f
  pharmacokinetic properties of, 35–38
  physical/chemical properties of,
    33–34
  recreational use of. *See* Recreational
    use of nitrous oxide
  safety of, 3, 39
  scavenging of, 173–174, 176–180
  second-gas effect of, 36, 38f
  sexual phenomena associated with,
    192–193
  solubility and partial pressure of, 83
  specific gravity of, 33
  storage of, 43–47, 45f
  titration of, 107–110
  toxicity of, 39
  utilization guidelines of, 193–194
Nitrous Oxide Abuse Task Force, 193
Nitrous Oxide Corporation, 43
Nitrous oxide/oxygen administration
  constant oxygen level technique of,
    129–130, 135b
  documentation of, 141, 142b, 143f,
    200
  education for, 198–199

Nitrous oxide/oxygen
  administration—cont'd
  ethical responsibilities in, 199–200
  guidelines for, 4, 200
  legal aspects of, 197–198
  licensure of, 197, 198
  overview of, 215
  patient participation in, 125–129
  patient positioning in, 119
  postoperative procedures in, 136–137
  preoperative unit preparation for,
    119–125
  principles of, 118–119
  technique for, 118–144
  titration technique in, 131–134, 133b,
    134f
Nitrous oxide/oxygen sedation
  acceptance of, 30
  age and, 202
  amnestic properties of, 29
  analgesic properties, 28
  anxiolytic properties of, 28–29
  asthma and, 202
  combined with other sedation
    methods, 14, 30–31
  compared to other sedation methods,
    28–30
    recovery from, 30
  customization of, 65
  design of, 63–65, 64–65f
  documentation of, 141, 142b, 143f,
    213
  eating before, 201
  economic benefits of, 70–74
  equipment for, 43–69. *See also*
    Equipment, sedation
  in ambulances, 151, 152f
  central vs. portable gas supply
    system, 65–66, 71–73, 72t
  evolution of, 10–15, 49–50
  resurgence of, 13
  in twentieth century, 13–15
  future trends in, 204
  history of, 6–10, 49–50
    discovery in, 6
    Dr. Colton's Grand Exhibition in, 9
    Horace Wells' experiment in, 9–10
    inhalation in, 6–8
    medical world in, 8–9
  hypnosuggestive properties of, 158
  income potential of, 71–74, 72b

Nitrous oxide/oxygen sedation—cont'd
insurance for, 202
manufacturers of, 49
multidisciplinary application of, 14,
149–160
nausea and vomiting from, 202
onset of action of, 29
open flame near, 201
oxycodone with, 202
patient costs for, 73–74
in pediatrics, 163–168. *See also*
Pediatrics, nitrous oxide/oxygen
sedation in
premedication with, 201
questions regarding, 201–203
signs and symptoms of, 111–117
titration of, 29–30
vital signs for, 101–102
intraoperative, 105
preoperative, 101–102
Nitrous oxide tanks
opening of, 120–121
pressure gauge indicator on, 120, 121f
Nociceptors, 16
Nonbreathing valve, 69
Nose, anatomy of, 77
Nutritional disorders, 95

O

Obstetrics/gynecology, 152–153
Occupational exposure
health hazards of, 171
inhalant abuse and, 186
prevention of, 180–181, 182b
Ophthalmic surgery, 94–95, 154
Ophthalmology, 154
Opioid system
activation of, 17
nitrous oxide effects on, 17
Oral sedation. *See* Premedication
Oropharynx, anatomy of, 77–78, 78f
Oscillating room fans, 180
Overexposure, prevention of, 180–181,
182b
Oversedation, signs and symptoms of,
114–117
Oximetry, pulse
in pediatric patients, 166
in recovery, 145
Oxycodone (Vicodin), with nitrous
oxide/oxygen sedation, 202

Oxygen
characteristics of, 34
cost of, 73
discovery of, 34
nitrous oxide and, 202
physical/chemical properties of,
34–35
preparation of, 34
saturation levels of, 84–86
storage of, 43–47, 45f, 48f, 49
titration of, 107–110
uses of, 35
Oxygen consumption, nitrous oxide
effect on, 90
Oxygen cylinders, 43–47, 45f, 48f, 49
pressure gauge reading of, 48f, 49
Oxygen fail-safe mechanism, 49, 66,
200
Oxygen flow, adjustment of, 125–127,
128b, 129
Oxygen flush button, 122, 123f, 128,
137
Oxygen tank
opening of, 120–121, 120f
pressure gauge indicator on, 120, 121f
Oxygenation, postoperative, 86, 138,
139f, 144
Oxymetry, pulse, indication for, 201
Ozone, nitrous oxide and, 34

P

Pain
assessment of, 18–19, 99–100
definition of, 16
foreign language words for, 19, 19b
incidence of, 16
preconceived expectations of, 20
principles of action in, 16–17
questions about, 99–100
reactions to, factors influencing, 17
Pain/anxiety management, 22–26, 23f,
28–29
decision making in, 26
history of, 8–10
individual biovariability in, 26
invasive, pharmacologic procedures
in, 24–26
noninvasive, nonpharmacologic
procedures for, 22–24, 23f
teaching of, guidelines for, 14
Pain intensity scales, 18–19, 19f, 100

Pain receptors, 16
Painful procedures, in children, nitrous oxide/oxygen sedation, 165
Parkinson's disease, 90
Partial pressure, 83
Partial pressure gradients, 35–36, 36f
Partition coefficients, 35
Patient(s)
 assessment of, 99–106
 comfort of, 119
 creating positive experiences for, 107, 108
 empathy toward, by health care professionals, 20
 feelings of, 119, 145
 instructions for. *See* Patient instruction(s)
 monitoring of, 101–102, 105, 118, 125, 128f, 136
 pediatric. *See* Children
 positioning of, 119
 questioning of, during recovery, 145
 reassurance of, 16, 17f, 28–29
 terminally ill. *See* Terminal illness
 transfer of, 151
Patient instruction(s), 119
 on breathing apparatus adjustments, 126
 on talking, 134
 during titration, 133
Patient preparation, 102
Patient risk
 ASA classification of, 100–101, 101b
 assessment of, 100–101
Pediatric patients. *See* Children
Pediatrics
 nitrous oxide/oxygen sedation, 158
 nitrous oxide/oxygen sedation in
  administration of, 166–167, 167f
  appointment length and, 168
  child development and, 163
  clinical application of, 163–168
  for dentistry, 163–164
  for emergency medicine, 164–165
  for gastrointestinal endoscopy, 165
  for painful procedures, 165
  patient considerations on, 165–166
  safety of, 167–168
  weight and, 166
Pentazocine addiction, withdrawal from, 156

Percutaneous biopsies, 156
Percutaneous cholangiography, 156
Peripheral neuropathy, 190, 191
Personal breathing zone, monitoring of, 180
Personal monitoring devices, 175–176
Pharynx, anatomy of, 77–79
Phobia, definition of, 20
Phobic individuals, nitrous oxide contraindicated in, 96
Physical Classification System, 100, 101b
Piaget's stages of child development, 163, 164t
Pin index safety system, 55, 55f, 56f
Piping system, central gas supply system, 51, 53
Piriform recess, 78, 79f
Pneumoencephalography, nitrous oxide effect on, 90
Pneumothorax
 caused by whippet chargers, 191
 nitrous oxide/oxygen sedation in, 92
Podiatry, 154
Polycythemia vera, 92
"Poppers," 186
Portable gas supply system, 53–55, 54f, 55f, 56–57f
 central gas supply system vs., 65–66, 71–73, 72t
 cost of, 65–66
 postoperative preparation of, 137
Porter, Gary, 50
Porter Instrument Company, 50
Positioning, of patient, 119
Positive-pressure oxygen hookup, 68f, 69
Postoperative oxygenation, 86, 138, 139f, 144
Practice guidelines, for nitrous oxide administration, 4, 200
Pregnancy, nitrous oxide effect on, 93–94, 173, 190
Prehospital care. *See* Emergency medicine
Premedication
 administered with nitrous oxide/oxygen sedation, 31
 with nitrous oxide/oxygen sedation, 201

Preoperative unit preparations, for nitrous oxide/oxygen administration, 119–125
  safety checks for, 119
Preoperative vital signs, 101–102
Pressure gauge indicator, 120, 121f
Pressure gauge reading of gas cylinders, 47, 48f, 49
Pressure hosing, portable gas supply system, 55, 57f
Pressure-reducing valves, central gas supply system, 53
Priestley, Joseph, 6, 34
Psychiatry, 155
Psychology, 155
Psychomotor ability, assessment of, 145
Psychotropic drugs, nitrous oxide contraindicated with, 96
Pulse
  monitoring of, 101, 125, 128f
  postoperative, 145
Pulse oximetry, 84–86, 85f
  indication for, 201
  in pediatric patients, 166
  in recovery, 145

Q

Quality of life
  in terminally ill patients, 159

R

Racing industry, nitrous oxide in, 43, 187
Radiology, 156–157
Rapid induction technique, in pediatric patients, 166
Record keeping. *See* Documentation
Recovery, 30, 144–148
  assessment of, 136, 145–147
  clinical studies of, 146–147
  postoperative symptoms in, 144
  principles of, 144
  psychologic and psychomotor effects of, 145
  return to work and, 201
Recovery time, 147
Recreational use of nitrous oxide, 185, 187–189
  adverse effects of, 190–192
  availability of, in food products, 188–189, 188f, 189f
  avoidance of, 199

Regulators
  central gas supply system, 53
  portable gas supply system, 55, 57f
Regulatory agencies and nitrous oxide packaging, 43
Regurgitation, silent, 91
  in oversedation, 117
Reproductive problems of occupational exposure to nitrous oxide, 173
Research, sex, 155
Reservoir bag(s), 58, 60, 60f, 69
  bulging of, 128, 128f
  collapse of, significance of, 203
  collapsing of, 128, 129f
  continuous inflation of, 128, 128f
  disinfection of, 138, 140
  filling of, 122–123, 124–125f
  inspection of, 119, 183
  in pediatric patients, 166
  purging contents of, 135, 136f
  as sign of conscious breathing, 134
Respiration
  anatomy and physiology of, 77–87
  monitoring of, 101–102, 125
Respiratory mechanism, physiology of, 81–86
Respiratory system
  anatomy and physiology of, 77–87
  nitrous oxide interaction with, 90–92
Respiratory zone, anatomy of, 81
Retardation, mental, 95
Rheumatic fever, 90
"Roller coaster" effect, 116
  in children, avoiding, 166
Room ventilation, assessment of, for nitrous oxide/oxygen administration, 119
Rubber hosing, sterilization of, 201

S

Safety
  of nitrous oxide, 3, 39
  of nitrous oxide/oxygen administration, 119
  of nitrous oxide/oxygen equipment, 66–69, 67–68f
  of nitrous oxide/oxygen sedation, in pediatric patients, 167–168
  of nitrous oxide/oxygen storage, 44, 46–47

Sales and Security Guidelines for the Safe Use/Handling of Nitrous Oxide, 193–194

Scales, for pain measurement, 18–19, 19f, 100

Scavenging, 173–174, 176–180
    problems with, 177

Scavenging mask system, 173–174

Scavenging nasal hoods, 61–62f, 63

Scavenging system, 177
    activation of, 121–122, 123f

Schizophrenia, 155

Seasonal allergies, 95

Second-gas effect, 36, 38f

Sedation. *See also* individual types of sedation
    appropriate minimal, signs and symptoms of, 111–114, 112b
    depth of, ASA continuum of, 21b
    equipment for, 63–69. *See also* Equipment, sedation
    history information on, 99
    mild, definition of, 21
    moderate
        discharge following, guidelines for, 147
        patients experiencing, management of, 86–87

Sedation-analgesia
    deep, definition of, 22
    moderate, definition of, 22

Sedative-hypnotics, nitrous oxide interacting with, 96

Seizure disorder, nitrous oxide effect on, 90

Semiconsciousness, nitrous oxide contraindicated during, 96

Sensory systems, 94

Sevoflurane, 39

Sex research, 155

Sex therapy, 155

Sexual impropriety, allegations of, against health professionals, 192–193

Sexual phenomena, associated with nitrous oxide, 192–193

Shock, nitrous oxide contraindicated during, 96

Sickle cell anemia, 92
    nitrous oxide/oxygen sedation and, 201

Silent regurgitation, 91
    in oversedation, 117

Silicon chip industry, nitrous oxide in, 43

Simpson, James, 11

Single-cylinder systems, in ambulances, 151

Sinusitis, nitrous oxide effect on, 90

Skin injuries, 151

Solubility, 35

Sophrology, combined with nitrous oxide/oxygen sedation, 30

Spasmodic torticollis, 160

Spectrophotometry, infrared, 174–175, 175f, 180
    equipment rental for, 202

Splinting, 151

Sterilization, 138–140, 141–142f
    of rubber hosing, 201

Stethoscope, pretracheal, 102, 103f

Stone, biliary, retrieval of, 156

Stroke, 90

Substance abuse, withdrawal from, 156

Subungual exostectomy, 154

Surgery, 90
    eye, 94–95, 154
    implant, ocular, 154

Suture removal, 151

Syndactylia, 15

T

Talking, during nitrous oxide/oxygen sedation, 134, 179–180

Talwin (pentazocine) addiction, withdrawal from, 156

Temporomandibular joint arthroscopy, bilateral, 156

TENS. *See* Transcutaneous electrical nerve stimulation (TENS)

Terminal illness, 159

Thiopental sodium, evolution of, 14

Thyroid gland dysfunction, 93

Tidal flow, 82

Tidal volume, 82, 83f
    adjustment of, 126–128, 127f, 128b, 128f, 129f

Time-weighted average dosimetry, in personal monitoring, 175, 176f

Titration, 29–30, 107–110, 133–135
    monitoring of, 134
    significance of, 108–110
    technique of, 131–134, 133b, 134f

Torticollis, spasmodic, 160
Tourette's syndrome, 160
Trace gases, scavenging of, 173–174
Trachea, anatomy of, 79–80, 80f
Transcutaneous electrical nerve
    stimulation (TENS), 24
Transfer, patient, 151
Trichloroethylene, 186
Trisomy 21, nitrous oxide/oxygen
    sedation and, 202
Tuberculosis, 92
Typewriter correction fluid, and
    inhalant abuse, 186

U

Ulcer, 93
Ultra flowmeter, 64
Upper airway, anatomy of, 77–79
Upper respiratory tract infections,
    90, 92
    nitrous oxide effect on, 90, 92
Urine testing, nitrous oxide detection in,
    189

V

Valleculae, 78, 79f
Venipuncture, 201
Ventilation, 179–180
    alveolar, 82
    minute, 82
    room, assessment of, for nitrous
        oxide/oxygen administration,
        119
Vicodin (oxycodone), with nitrous
    oxide/oxygen sedation, 202
Visceral arteriography, 156

Vital signs
    assessment of, 101–102, 125, 128f
    intraoperative, 105
    monitoring of, 101–102
    for nitrous oxide/oxygen sedation,
        101–102
    preoperative, 101–102
    significance of, in preprocedural
        evaluation, 101–102
Vitamin B_{12}, nitrous oxide effect on, 39,
    172, 190
Vitamin B_{12} supplements, in pregnant
    women, 190
Vomiting, in oversedation, 117, 202
Vomitus, aspiration of, in moderate
    sedation, management of, 87

W

Wart removal, 151
Waste gas removal, during nitrous
    oxide/oxygen administration, 119
Weight, nitrous oxide/oxygen sedation
    in children and, 166
Wells, Horace, 9–10, 10f, 11–12, 12f, 49
Whippet chargers, adverse effects of, 191
Whippets, as source of nitrous oxide
    abuse, 188–189, 188f
Whipping cream propellant, as source of
    nitrous oxide abuse, 188–189,
    188f, 189f
Withdrawal, from addiction, 156
Wound debridement, 151

Y

Yoke stand, portable gas supply system,
    51–52, 53–55, 54–55f